dairy free

lactose-free
DIET PLAN
FOR CHILDREN & ADULTS

So now you will Lots of Love From Jenny (Mar '06)
maybe be impressing   xxxx
me even more with
your culinary skills!
Hope you find some good .
ideas.

dairy free

lactose-free

DIET PLAN
FOR CHILDREN & ADULTS

carolyn humphries

foulsham
LONDON • NEW YORK • TORONTO • SYDNEY

foulsham

The Publishing House, Bennetts Close,
Cippenham, Slough, Berks, SL1 5AP, England

Cover photograph © The Image Bank

Consultant dietician:
Tanya Wright, Senior Dietician, Stoke Mandeville Hospital

ISBN 0-572-02683-8

Printed in Great Britain by St. Edmundsbury Press, Bury St. Edmunds, Suffolk

CONTENTS

Introduction   7

All you Need to Know about Milk Allergies   9

Your General Health and Well-being   15

Notes on the Recipes   17

Feel the Difference in Just Seven Days   19

Breakfasts   23

Soups, Starters and Snacks   39

Fish and Vegetable Main Courses   61

Meat and Poultry Main Courses   87

Desserts   119

Children's Specials   137

Breads, Biscuits, Cakes and Pastries   157

Sauces, Dressings, Cheeses and Creams   177

Index   187

INTRODUCTION

Over the last 15 years, food allergies have become more widely recognised and when children or adults begin to suffer problems of one kind or another, the cause is often traced to dairy products. There are two types of problem: lactose intolerance and cows' milk protein allergy.

These problems frequently start in infancy and can mean a difficult time not only for the children, but also for their parents, who have to enforce a dairy-free diet and explain why the children can't eat the biscuits (cookies), cakes, ice cream or milk shakes their friends and siblings are enjoying. Unfortunately, however, this is not the only problem as an allergy can start at any time of life. Many people have to learn to cope with an allergy that means they have to face the prospect of making fairly major changes in their dietary habits.

This book is designed to make that change as easy and stress-free as possible. To start with, I have explained clearly and simply what the conditions of lactose intolerance and cows' milk protein allergy are, and how the various symptoms can manifest themselves, so you can fully understand the problems and what you need to do about them.

I have created a whole range of delicious dairy-free alternative recipes for many popular foods – from the smoothest chocolate milkshake to the tangiest of lemon cheesecakes. There are dishes for every meal of the day and a whole range of sumptuous snacks too. There is even a special section on children's favourites that all kids will love whether they have a milk allergy or not! All the recipes in the book are suitable both for those with cows' milk protein allergy and lactose intolerance. So with the help of this book, your family's diet can remain as interesting, nourishing and varied as if you did not have to cope with an allergy in the family.

ALL YOU NEED TO KNOW ABOUT MILK ALLERGIES

LACTOSE INTOLERANCE

Lactose is a disaccharide – a natural sugar – found in human milk and the milk of other mammals. During normal digestion, an enzyme called lactase breaks down the lactose in the small intestine, making it into simple sugars – glucose and galactose – so the body can absorb it. If our bodies do not produce enough lactase, the lactose passes, unprocessed, into the large intestine where the naturally present bacteria feed on it, giving off gas and toxins, and causing pain, bloating, flatulence and diarrhoea.

This condition is usually inherited and is most common amongst adolescents and adults, but in rare cases a child is born without any ability to make lactase.

Some races – particularly those from South-east Asia, the Middle East, parts of Africa and India – are more susceptible because they do not normally drink milk after infancy, so the body stops producing the lactase enzyme altogether. Some of these sufferers find that if they persist with drinking milk on a regular basis, the body begins to produce the enzyme again and their problems are overcome. The condition can also be brought on temporarily by malnutrition or gastrointestinal infections or because another disease has damaged the lining of the small intestine.

The amount of milk needed to cause the symptoms of the intolerance varies widely. Some people with enzyme deficiency can drink as much as a glass of milk a day without any problems, sometimes more if mixed with other foods; others must avoid it altogether. Your specialist will advise you on your particular condition and then it will be a case of trial and error to find out how much you can consume without reacting.

Hard cheese and fermented milk products such as yoghurt can often be eaten by people who are lactose-intolerant without side-effects. But to make the recipes in this book suitable for all sufferers, I have eliminated all dairy products. If you find that you can tolerate some additional products, you can vary the recipes to suit your own circumstances.

COWS' MILK PROTEIN ALLERGY

This is a condition in which the body reacts adversely to the protein in cows' milk. The range of possible symptoms is extensive, including a blocked-up or runny nose, wheezing, coughing, diarrhoea, skin rashes and lumps, eczema, a swollen stomach, vomiting, headaches, and even hyperactivity amongst toddlers. The allergy is particularly prevalent among infants and young children but can occur at any age. It is most common in families with a history of other allergies, such as asthma or eczema. In very severe cases, it can cause anaphylactic shock, but this is very rare.

In young babies, the problem is fairly easily detected. Symptoms will begin soon after the introduction of cows' milk formula. A baby may cry a great deal, become listless, suffer from colic and fail to thrive. If you suspect this problem in your baby, you should consult your health visitor or GP immediately. It is a fairly common problem, affecting about two babies in every 100. Some particularly sensitive breast-fed babies may develop an intolerance through milk the mother has digested, so it is recommended that the mother has to change her diet. Fortunately, many children outgrow the condition by the age of five and it usually only continues if the child also suffers from other allergies.

In adulthood, a cows' milk protein allergy is more difficult to detect. Reaction usually occurs from 45 minutes to 20 hours after consumption, and as the sufferer may have other allergies that produce similar symptoms, allergy tests by the GP or consultant will be needed to confirm the diagnosis.

A FEW WORDS OF WARNING

This book is not a substitute for professional medical advice. No one should go on any kind of exclusion diet without first consulting a doctor, so if you suspect you have an allergy to cows' milk, do not simply cut it out of your diet immediately. Milk is a highly valuable food, providing not only protein but fat, carbohydrate, essential minerals (particularly calcium for healthy teeth and bones and zinc to help fight infection and for growth), and A, B-group and C vitamins. For this reason, you should never cut out all dairy products from your diet unless your doctor advises you that it is absolutely necessary. Your specialist may suggest you exclude them for a short while, then try introducing them gradually to see how much can be tolerated.

The above advice applies particularly to children.

If you do have to cut out dairy products altogether, this can cause a deficiency of certain vitamins and minerals, particularly calcium. Check with your specialist whether you need a vitamin and mineral supplement and make sure you eat other foods that are rich in calcium (see Healthy Bones and Teeth, page 16).

Do not assume that you can use soya milk as an alternative. People with severe allergic reactions may also react to soya products. If this is the case, you must consult your specialist for dietary alternatives.

Above all, don't try to use this book as the basis for a do-it-yourself diet. Without professional advice, you will probably still be eating foods that contain hidden sources of milk protein or lactose – they are found in the most unexpected foods.

ALTERNATIVES TO DAIRY PRODUCTS

Fortunately, there are now many products on the market that can be used instead of dairy products and they are readily available in major supermarkets. Other ranges of lactose-free products, such as rice and nut milks, are available at health food shops, at a price.

- Soya milk is the obvious choice for most people as a substitute for cows' milk (but see above). I recommend one sweetened with apple juice (which is far more palatable) and enriched with calcium.
- There are also various oat milks in powder and liquid form. I particularly like a Swedish oat drink, which has a slightly nutty taste that complements cereals very well. Use this instead of soya milk in any of the recipes if you prefer.
- Some people with milk allergies can tolerate goats' and sheep's milk and cheeses, and water buffalo Mozzarella. However, to make the recipes in this book suitable for all sufferers, I have not used any of them. But if you find that you can tolerate any of these – or hard cheeses such as Cheddar or Parmesan – then do use them. You may also find that you can tolerate Edam, Brie and blue cheese. Failing that, there is a large range of soya cheeses.
- Pure soya spread is, in my opinion, the best alternative to butter or margarine for cooking. You can also use any nut, vegetable or olive oils, but do make sure that there are no 'hidden' dairy ingredients. There are many dairy-free spreads now available in supermarkets.
- White vegetable fat is also useful, particularly for making pastry (paste).
- Soya Dream is an excellent commercial UHT substitute for single (light) cream, and soya yoghurt also tastes very good.
- Tofu (fermented bean curd) is very useful. Silken tofu is creamy and good for dips, sauces and toppings. Firm tofu can be marinated and used instead of cheese or meat.

READ THE LABELS FOR HIDDEN MILK PRODUCTS

Apart from the obvious dairy ingredients – such as butter, milk and any type of cream – milk products appear in numerous guises in commercial products, from batters to biscuits (cookies), and margarines to medicines. Watch out for the following in lists of ingredients (those marked with an asterisk may or may not contain milk products):

- Butter as fat, flavouring, oil or solids
- Caramel colouring*
- Casein, hydrolised casein, rennet casein
- Caseinates (ammonium, calcium, magnesium, potassium, sodium)
- Curds
- Dried milk (non-fat milk powder)
- Dry milk solids
- Flavouring*
- High-protein flour*
- Hydrolised milk protein
- Lactalbumin, lactalbumin phosphate
- Lactate
- Lactoferrin
- Lactoglobulin
- Lactose
- Milk derivative-fat/solids
- Natural flavouring*
- Non-fat milk/milk solids
- Opta (fat replacer)
- Simplesse (fat replacer)
- Solids
- Soured (dairy sour) cream solids/milk solids
- Whey, delactosed whey, demineralised whey, sweet whey powder, whey powder, whey protein concentrate, whey solids

MILK WHERE YOU'D LEAST EXPECT IT

Milk can also be found in many commercially prepared foods – and some of them are quite surprising! Here is a list of those you should be wary of because they may contain milk in one form or another.
- Biscuits (cookies)
- Bread – in any shape or form
- Breakfast cereals, including muesli
- Candies and other sweets
- Canned and packet soups
- Chocolate – plain (semi-sweet) as well as milk and white
- Crisps (chips), especially flavoured varieties
- Crumb- or batter-coated fish, chicken, etc.

- Custards
- Crackers
- Doughnuts
- Hot dogs
- Instant hot drinks
- Instant mashed potato
- Margarine
- Pancakes
- Pickles, sauces and relishes
- Pie fillings
- Pizzas
- Processed meats, including ham
- Salad cream, salad dressings
- Sausages
- Scones (biscuits)
- Stock cubes
- Waffles

Remember to take care with home-made produce too – even that delicious jam or marmalade your neighbour gives you may have had a knob of butter added.

PROBLEMS WITH PILLS

More than 20 per cent of prescription drugs and around 6 per cent of over-the-counter medicines contain lactose. But the quantities used are so small that they should only affect you if you have a very severe allergy or lactose intolerance. They should not affect those with a milk protein allergy. However, check with your doctor or pharmacist before taking anything, to be on the safe side. If you do react to a medicine, it is far more likely to be the drug itself that is upsetting you than the milk sugar it contains.

YOUR GENERAL HEALTH AND WELL-BEING

Everyone needs a healthy balanced diet. Every day you need to have foods from all the main food groups but in differing proportions.

Carbohydrates for energy: There are two types of carbohydrate: complex and simple. Complex carbohydrates are all the starchy foods you eat such as bread, pasta, rice, cereals and potatoes. Eat plenty of these for energy. Simple carbohydrates are sugars. They are found naturally in many foods but are also manufactured commercially in many forms: all the granular sugars, syrups, black treacle (molasses) and honey. You get quite enough for a balanced diet in natural foods, so all the extra you sprinkle on or put in biscuits, cakes and puddings just piles on extra, unnecessary calories. So don't overdo it.

Proteins for body growth and repair: Dairy products are one of the main sources, and since you are excluding them from your diet you have to find alternatives. Choose from lean meat, poultry, game, fish, eggs, pulses – dried peas, beans and lentils – and manufactured vegetable proteins such as soya protein, tofu (bean curd) and Quorn. Eat two or three small portions a day.

Vitamins and minerals for general well-being: The best sources of these are fruit and vegetables, ideally fresh, but those frozen or canned in water or natural juice are also fine. Eat at least five portions a day.

Fibre for healthy body functioning: Fibre is simply the bulky substance in food that passes through the system and keeps the muscles of your digestive system well exercised! If you don't have enough fibre in your diet, your gut becomes a proverbial couch potato and can't do its job properly. Eat plenty of fruit and vegetables, cereals, nuts, seeds and dried fruit. Leave the skins on potatoes and fruit, where appropriate.

Fat for warmth and energy and to protect the skin, muscles and organs: Although we should not eat too much fat in our diet, especially if we have a sedentary lifestyle, some fat is essential. All the fat you need is found naturally in foods so eat naturally fatty foods sparingly and keep added fat – in the form of oils or whatever spreads you choose – to the minimum.

HEALTHY TEETH AND BONES

Calcium is vital for growth and to maintain healthy teeth and bones. In a diet that contains little or no milk, it can be tricky to get enough. Calcium-enriched soya milk will help, but it is also important to eat other foods rich in this mineral. These are:
- Baked beans
- Bread – check that it's milk-free
- Dried fruit
- Eggs
- Fish and seafood – try to include canned salmon, pilchards and sardines with soft, edible bones as these are excellent sources of calcium
- Green vegetables
- Nuts

Check with your doctor in case you need a supplement too. Calcium is particularly important for children and lactating or post-menopausal women. Low levels of calcium in the elderly may also increase the risk of osteoporosis.

EXERCISE

It may not be anything to do with your diet, but regular, sensible exercise is an important part of a healthy lifestyle. Try to walk rather than taking the car, send the children out into the garden with a football instead of putting on a video, and make exercise a part of your daily life.

NOTES ON THE RECIPES

- All ingredients are given in imperial, metric and American measures. Follow one set only in a recipe. American terms are given in brackets.

- All spoon measures are level: 1 tsp = 5 ml;
  1 tbsp = 15 ml

- Eggs are medium unless otherwise stated.

- Always wash, peel, core and seed, if necessary, fresh produce before use.

- Seasoning and the use of strongly flavoured ingredients such as garlic or chillies are very much a matter of personal taste. Adjust seasonings to suit your own palate and digestion.

- I have used soya milk in all the recipes, but you can use oat drink instead, if you prefer. If you can take lactose-reduced milk, then do use that.

- Always use fresh herbs unless dried are specifically called for. If you wish to substitute dried for fresh, use only half the quantity or less as they are very pungent. Frozen, chopped varieties have a better flavour than the dried ones.

- All can sizes are approximate as they vary from brand to brand. For example, if I call for a 400 g/14 oz/ large can of tomatoes and yours is a 397 g can – that's fine.

- Cooking times are approximate and should be used as a guide only. Always check that food is thoroughly cooked through before serving.

- I have avoided all use of cows' milk products. However, if you can tolerate hard cheese, like Parmesan or Cheddar, or ordinary yoghurt, or goats' or sheep's milk products, do use them.

FEEL THE DIFFERENCE IN JUST SEVEN DAYS

This is just to show you how delicious your new diet can be. I have given different fruit breakfast choices and different tea-time treats every day but, of course, in reality you are more likely to use up a carton of juice or make one batch of biscuits (cookies) or one cake at a time.

DAY ONE

Breakfast	Glass of orange juice Honey Fruit and Nut Crunch (page 27) Tea or coffee
Lunch	Mighty Minestrone (page 43) French bread A nectarine
Teatime treat	Chocolate Digestive (page 151)
Dinner	Steak Strips Sizzle with Crunchy Noodles (page 90) Apricot Fool (page 125)

DAY TWO

Breakfast	Glass of grapefruit juice Fresh Blueberry Muffin (page 38) Tea or coffee
Lunch	Bruschetta (page 52) A banana
Teatime treat	Ginger Crumblie (page 176)
Dinner	Sage and Onion Sausage Toad with Carrot Gravy (page 100) Chocolate Ice (page 121)

DAY THREE

Breakfast	Slice of melon Kipper and Egg Scramble (page 33) Tea or coffee
Lunch	Peanut Rarebit (page 57) Soya yoghurt with honey
Teatime treat	Slice of Everyday Fruit Cake (page 167)
Dinner	Spicy Prawn Fajitas (page 70) Lemon Cheesecake (page 123)

DAY FOUR

Breakfast	Glass of tomato juice French Toast (page 35) Tea or coffee
Lunch	Rich Tomato and Rice Soup (page 41) An apple
Teatime treat	Sweet Yoghurt Scone (page 164) with soya spread and jam (conserve)
Dinner	Smoky Caesar Salad (page 112) Peach Filo Tarts (page 126)

DAY FIVE

Breakfast	Glass of orange juice Tofu, Apple and Blackberry Kissel (page 25) Slice of toast, soya spread and honey Tea or coffee
Lunch	Spiced Banana and Corn Toppers (page 51) Soya yoghurt with raisins
Teatime treat	Muesli Cookie (page 175)
Dinner	Savoury Egg Pasta (page 74) Cherries with Kirsch Zabaglione (page 134)

DAY SIX

Breakfast	Glass of grapefruit juice Creamy Golden Trickle Porridge (page 28) Slice of toast, soya spread and marmalade
Lunch	Grilled Marinated Tofu on Toast (page 55) An orange
Teatime treat	Slice of Jam and 'Cream' Sponge (page 165)
Dinner	Monkfish Tabbouleh (page 62) Almost Tiramisu (page 132)

DAY SEVEN

Breakfast	Slice of melon Potato Cakes with Bacon and Eggs (page 31) Soya Breakfast Roll (page 37) with soya spread and marmalade Tea or coffee
Lunch	Stuffed Pot Roast Chicken (page 114) Bread and Jam Pudding (page 122)
Teatime treat	Maid of Honour (page 171)
Dinner	Creamy Mushroom Soup (page 40) A pear

BREAKFASTS

Breakfast is, arguably, the most important meal of the day. If you don't like the taste of plain soya milk, try putting apple or orange juice on your cereal – it's delicious, especially on muesli. Also, as I've said before, if you are lactose intolerant, you may well be able to eat ordinary yoghurt, which is also great on cereal (and soya yoghurt tastes fine). But here are some delicious, and more exciting, breakfast ideas for you to enjoy. Always have a glass of fruit juice or a piece of fresh fruit as part of your breakfast: it will help absorb any iron in your cereal as well as giving you added vitamin C.

Banana Breakfast Whip

SERVES 1

1 large ripe banana

200 ml/7 fl oz/scant 1 cup soya milk

15 ml/1 tbsp clear honey

15 ml/1 tbsp oat bran

1 Purée the banana in a blender or food processor.

2 Add the remaining ingredients and blend until thick and frothy.

3 Pour into a glass and serve immediately.

Banana, Strawberry and Almond Wake-up

SERVES 1

1 ripe banana

6 ripe strawberries

30 ml/2 tbsp ground almonds

150 ml/¼ pt/⅔ cup apple juice

150 ml/¼ pt/⅔ cup soya milk

Ice cubes

1 Purée the banana and strawberries in a blender or food processor.

2 Add the ground almonds and apple juice and run the machine again.

3 Add the soya milk and blend once more. Pour into a glass, top with ice cubes and serve.

Tofu Apple and Blackberry Kissel

*This can be made in advance and then reheated, if liked,
before serving*

SERVES 4

---

1 large cooking (tart) apple, sliced

100 g/4 oz blackberries

Finely grated rind and juice of 1 orange

Light brown sugar, to taste

150 ml/¼ pt/⅔ cup water

100 g/4 oz/½ cup firm tofu

10 ml/2 tsp cornflour (cornstarch) or potato flour

*60 ml/4 tbsp silken tofu and 30 ml/2 tbsp toasted
flaked (slivered) almonds, to serve*

1 Put the apple and blackberries in a saucepan with the orange rind and juice, about 30 ml/2 tbsp sugar and half the water.

2 Bring to the boil, reduce the heat and simmer gently until the fruit is pulpy.

3 Purée in a blender or food processor with the firm tofu and pass through a sieve (strainer) to remove the seeds, if liked, before returning to the saucepan.

4 Blend the cornflour or potato flour with the remaining water and stir into the purée.

5 Bring to the boil and cook for 2 minutes, stirring. Taste and add more sugar, if necessary.

6 Serve hot or cold, topped with the silken tofu and almonds.

Breakfast Compôte

225 g/8 oz/1⅓ cups mixed dried fruit salad

600 ml/1 pt/2½ cups water

2.5 cm/1 in piece of cinnamon stick

1 clove

Clear honey (optional)

Soya yoghurt, to serve

1 Soak the dried fruit in the water in a saucepan for several hours or overnight.

2 Add the cinnamon and clove and bring to the boil. Reduce the heat, part-cover and simmer gently for 20 minutes or until completely tender but with the fruits still holding their shape. Discard the spices.

3 Sweeten, if liked, with a little honey.

4 Serve warm or cold topped with soya yoghurt.

Honey Fruit and Nut Crunch

Once made, this can be stored in an airtight container.

SERVES 6–8

75 g/3 oz/¾ cup rolled oats

75 g/3 oz/¾ cup millet flakes

90 ml/6 tbsp chopped mixed nuts

45 ml/3 tbsp sultanas (golden raisins)

60 ml/4 tbsp clear honey

Soya milk, to serve

1 Toss the oats and millet flakes with the nuts in a heavy-based frying pan (skillet) over a gentle heat until just turning golden.

2 Add the sultanas and honey and toss to coat for 30 seconds until you can smell the sugar but the mixture is not burning.

3 Immediately turn out on to a sheet of non-stick baking parchment and leave to cool.

4 Serve in bowls with soya milk.

Creamy Golden Trickle Porridge

100 g/4 oz/1 cup rolled oats

A pinch of salt

300 ml/½ pt/1¼ cups water

300 ml/½ pt/1¼ cups soya milk

60 ml/4 tbsp Soya Dream (see page 12)

60 ml/4 tbsp golden (light corn) syrup

1 Put the oats in a non-stick saucepan with the salt and gradually blend in the water and milk. Bring to the boil, stirring.

2 Reduce the heat and simmer, stirring, for 5 minutes until thick and creamy.

3 Spoon into warm bowls, top each with a spoonful of Soya Dream and trickle the golden syrup all over the surface.

Tropical Oats

600 ml/1 pt/2½ cups water

65 g/2½ oz/scant ¾ cup medium oatmeal

50 g/2 oz/⅓ cup stoned (pitted) dried dates, chopped

50 g/2 oz/⅓ cup raisins

50 g/2 oz creamed coconut, cut into pieces

Light brown sugar and soya milk, to serve

1 Bring the water to the boil in a non-stick saucepan.

2 Add the oatmeal in a steady stream, stirring all the time. Bring back to the boil, reduce the heat as low as possible, and simmer, stirring occasionally, for 10 minutes.

3 Add the fruit and creamed coconut and keep stirring until the coconut melts. Thin with a little soya milk, if necessary.

4 Spoon into bowls, sprinkle with a very little brown sugar and serve with soya milk.

Summer Porridge

You can make this the night before and cover with a circle of wet greaseproof (waxed) paper to prevent a skin forming, then reheat for breakfast.

SERVES 4

100 g/4 oz strawberries, sliced

100 g/4 oz raspberries

30 ml/2 tbsp caster (superfine) sugar

600 ml/1 pt/2½ cups water

50 g/2 oz/⅓ cup semolina (cream of wheat)

Lemon juice (optional)

1 Reserve a few pieces of fruit for decoration. Purée the remainder in a blender or food processor, then pass through a sieve (strainer) into a saucepan to remove the seeds.

2 Stir the sugar and water into the fruit and bring to the boil. Pour in the semolina in a thin stream, whisking all the time with a wire whisk.

3 Bring back to the boil, reduce the heat and simmer gently for 10 minutes, stirring occasionally, until thick and smooth. Taste and sharpen with a little lemon juice, if liked.

4 Serve hot, decorated with the reserved berries.

Potato Cakes with Bacon and Eggs

SERVES 4

60 ml/4 tbsp sunflower oil

1 onion, finely chopped

2 rashers (slices) of streaky bacon, rinded and chopped

1 large potato, grated

A pinch of dried mixed herbs

Salt and freshly ground black pepper

15 ml/1 tbsp plain (all-purpose) flour

5 eggs

1 Heat 10 ml/2 tsp of the oil in a frying pan (skillet) and add the onion and bacon. Fry (sauté), stirring, for 2 minutes.

2 Tip into a bowl and mix with the potato, herbs, a little salt and pepper and the flour.

3 Beat one of the eggs and stir into the potato mixture.

4 Heat 30 ml/2 tbsp of the remaining oil in the frying pan and fry spoonfuls of the mixture for about 3 minutes until golden brown underneath. Turn over and cook the other sides for a further 2 minutes or until cooked through. Drain on kitchen paper (paper towels) and keep warm.

5 Heat the remaining oil in the pan and fry the four remaining eggs until cooked to your liking.

6 Slide on to warm plates and serve with the potato cakes.

Herby Mushroom and Egg Cups with Crunchy Bacon

SERVES 4
4 large open-cup mushrooms
15 g/½ oz/1 tbsp soya spread
Salt and freshly ground black pepper
5 ml/1 tsp chopped fresh oregano
5 ml/1 tsp chopped fresh parsley
5 ml/1 tsp snipped fresh chives
60 ml/4 tbsp water
4 rashers (slices) of streaky bacon, rinded
15 ml/1 tbsp lemon juice
4 eggs
Dairy-free bread and soya spread, to serve

1 Peel the mushrooms. Remove, trim and chop the stalks.

2 Melt the soya spread in a frying pan (skillet), add the mushrooms, gill-sides up, and sprinkle the chopped stalks in the cups. Fry (sauté) for 2 minutes, then season each with a little salt and pepper and the herbs. Pour the water around, cover tightly with a lid or foil, and cook over a gentle heat for about 5 minutes until tender.

3 Meanwhile, grill (broil) the bacon until crisp, then snip into pieces with scissors.

4 Bring a frying pan of water to the boil and add the lemon juice. Reduce the heat so that the water is just simmering. Break the eggs one at a time into a cup and slide into the simmering water. Cover and poach for about 3 minutes until cooked to your liking.

5 Transfer the mushrooms to warm plates with any juices left in the pan. Lift the eggs out of the water with a slotted spoon, drain well and place on top of the mushrooms. Sprinkle with the bacon and serve straight away with bread and soya spread.

Kipper and Egg Scramble

SERVES 4

2 kipper fillets, skinned and cut into bite-sized pieces

Boiling water

6 eggs

45 ml/3 tbsp soya milk

Salt and freshly ground black pepper

A good knob of soya spread, plus extra for spreading

4 slices of dairy-free granary bread

15 ml/1 tbsp chopped fresh parsley

1 Put the kipper pieces in a shallow dish. Pour over just enough water to cover, place a lid or foil over and leave to stand for 5 minutes.

2 Meanwhile, beat the eggs and soya milk in a saucepan. Add a pinch of salt, a good grinding of pepper and the knob of soya spread.

3 Cook over a fairly gentle heat, stirring all the time until the mixture is scrambled but still creamy. Do not allow to boil or the mixture will curdle.

4 Drain the kipper pieces thoroughly and stir into the eggs.

5 Meanwhile, toast the bread and spread with soya spread. Place on warm plates. Pile the egg and kipper mixture on top and sprinkle with chopped parsley.

Brioches

Make these in advance, then serve warm or cold for breakfast.

MAKES 12

---

250 g/9 oz/2¼ cups plain (all-purpose) flour

2.5 ml/½ tsp salt

15 ml/1 tbsp caster (superfine) sugar

10 ml/2 tsp easy-blend dried yeast

2 whole eggs

2 egg yolks

50 g/2 oz/¼ cup soya spread, melted

60 ml/4 tbsp hand-hot water

Sunflower oil, for greasing

Soya spread and cherry jam (conserve), to serve

---

1 Mix the flour, salt, sugar and yeast in a large bowl and make a well in the centre.

2 Beat the eggs and egg yolks together and reserve 10 ml/2 tsp for glazing.

3 Pour the eggs and melted soya spread into the flour and work with a wooden spoon, then draw together with your hand, adding the water and kneading to form a smooth, sticky dough.

4 Cover the bowl with lightly greased clingfilm (plastic wrap) and leave in a warm place for about 45 minutes or until the dough has doubled in bulk.

5 Knock back (punch down) and knead gently on a lightly floured surface.

6 Divide the dough into three equal pieces. Cut each of two of the pieces into six, making 12 small pieces, and roll into balls. Place in the greased sections of a tartlet tin (patty pan) or separate brioche tins.

7   Roll the remaining piece of dough into 12 small balls. Make a hollow in the centre of each ball in the tins and gently press one of the small balls into each hollow. Leave in a warm place for 15–20 minutes until doubled in bulk again.

8   Brush lightly with the reserved beaten egg and bake in a preheated oven at 230°C/450°F/gas mark 8 for about 10 minutes until golden and the bases sound hollow when turned out and tapped. Turn out on to a wire rack and leave to cool. Serve with soya spread and cherry jam.

French Toast

SERVES 4

1 egg

30 ml/2 tbsp soya milk

4 slices of dairy-free white bread, crusts removed

25 g/1 oz/2 tbsp soya spread

30 ml/2 tbsp sunflower oil

20 ml/4 tsp caster (superfine) sugar

5 ml/1 tsp ground cinnamon

1   Beat the egg with the soya milk in a shallow dish.

2   Cut the bread into triangles and dip in the egg mixture until soaked on both sides.

3   Heat the soya spread and oil in a frying pan (skillet). Fry (sauté) the bread on both sides until golden brown. Drain on kitchen paper (paper towels).

4   Mix the sugar and cinnamon together and dust all over both sides of the eggy bread. Serve straight away.

English Breakfast Muffins

To serve these fresh for breakfast, prepare to step 6, then store in the fridge overnight, ready to cook in the morning.

MAKES 6

---

100 g/4 oz/1 cup strong plain (bread) flour

75 g/3 oz/¾ cup plain (all-purpose) flour

2.5 ml/½ tsp salt

10 ml/2 tsp easy-blend dried yeast

10 g/¼ oz/2 tsp soya spread, plus extra for spreading

60 ml/4 tbsp soya milk

About 60 ml/4 tbsp hand-hot water

Cornflour (cornstarch), for dusting

Sunflower oil, for greasing

Honey, to serve

1 Sift the flours and salt into a bowl. Stir in the yeast.

2 Melt the soya spread with the milk. Cool to hand-hot, then, using a wooden spoon, stir into the flour with enough water to form a sticky dough, then draw together with your hand, kneading until smooth and elastic.

3 Cover the bowl with lightly greased clingfilm (plastic wrap) and leave in a warm place for about 1 hour until doubled in bulk.

4 Knock back (punch down) the dough and divide into six pieces.

5 Dust your hands with cornflour, then shape the dough into balls and place on a baking (cookie) sheet, dusted with more cornflour.

6 Cover with clingfilm, dusted with more cornflour, and leave in a warm place for about 40 minutes until well risen again.

7 Heat a heavy-based frying pan (skillet) very lightly oiled (or use two if you want to cook all the muffins at once). Carefully transfer three muffins to the pan and cook gently for about 8 minutes on each side until a very pale golden brown and cooked through.

8 Serve split and spread with soya spread and honey. They can also be split and toasted.

Soya Breakfast Rolls

MAKES 10

1 quantity of Milk Bread dough (see page 160)

A little sunflower oil, for greasing

Soya milk, for glazing

Soya spread and marmalade, to serve

1 Make up the bread dough. When knocked back (punched down), knead gently on a lightly floured surface.

2 Shape into 10 oval rolls and make a few snips in the top of each with kitchen scissors. Place on a lightly greased baking (cookie) sheet. Leave in a warm place for about 20 minutes until doubled in bulk.

3 Brush with a little soya milk to glaze, and bake towards the top of a preheated oven at 220°C/425°F/ gas mark 7 for about 15 minutes until golden and the bases sound hollow when tapped.

4 Serve warm or cold with soya spread and marmalade.

Fresh Blueberry Muffins

Ring the changes with other soft fruits such as raspberries or chopped apricots.

MAKES 12

---

275 g/10 oz/2½ cups self-raising (self-rising) flour

5 ml/1 tsp baking powder

Finely grated rind of ½ orange

100 g/4 oz/½ cup caster (superfine) sugar

1 egg

150 ml/¼ pt/⅔ cup soya yoghurt

100 ml/3½ fl oz/scant ½ cup soya milk

60 ml/4 tbsp sunflower oil

175 g/6 oz blueberries

1 Line a deep tartlet tin (patty pan) or muffin tin with paper cake cases (cupcake papers).

2 Sift the flour and baking powder together into a bowl and stir in the orange rind and sugar.

3 Lightly beat the egg, yoghurt, milk and oil together and beat into the flour mixture.

4 Fold in the blueberries with a metal spoon.

5 Spoon the mixture into the prepared tins and bake in a preheated oven at 200°C/400°F/gas mark 6 for about 20–25 minutes until risen, golden and firm to the touch.

6 Transfer to a wire rack to cool. Serve warm or cold.

SOUPS, STARTERS AND SNACKS

Soups make wonderful, nutritious light
meals as well as being the perfect
opener for a more formal occasion.
However, many, especially the creamed
ones, usually contain dairy produce –
but not my versions! You will find that,
accompanied with some fresh bread,
many of the starters in this chapter
make delicious lunches or suppers,
which makes them doubly useful. The
snacks here could be used for packed
lunches, as a midday nibble or a TV
supper. They are designed to be easy to
make, easy to eat and, of course, totally
delicious and dairy-free.

Creamy Mushroom Soup

SERVES 4

50 g/2 oz/¼ cup soya spread

225 g/8 oz small button mushrooms, finely chopped

45 ml/3 tbsp plain (all-purpose) flour

600 ml/1 pt/2½ cups lactose-free chicken stock

150 ml/¼ pt/⅔ cup soya milk

1 bay leaf

45 ml/3 tbsp Soya Dream (see page 12)

Salt and freshly ground black pepper

15 ml/1 tbsp chopped fresh parsley, to garnish

1 Heat the spread in a saucepan and fry (sauté) the mushrooms gently for 2 minutes, stirring until softened but not browned.

2 Stir in the flour and cook for 2 minutes, stirring.

3 Remove from the heat and gradually blend in the stock and milk. Return to the heat and bring to the boil, stirring. Add the bay leaf.

4 Part-cover the pan, reduce the heat and simmer gently for 10 minutes. Discard the bay leaf. Stir in 30 ml/ 2 tbsp of the Soya Dream and season to taste.

5 Ladle into warm bowls, top each with a swirl of the remaining Soya Dream and sprinkle with parsley.

Rich Tomato and Rice Soup

Give this a Mediterranean flavour by adding 30 ml/2 tbsp chopped fresh basil just before serving.

SERVES 6

1 onion, chopped

2 carrots, chopped

1 celery stick, chopped

25 g/1 oz/2 tbsp soya spread

45 ml/3 tbsp plain (all-purpose) flour

1.2 litres/2 pts/5 cups lactose-free chicken stock

700 g/1½ lb tomatoes, skinned and chopped

15 ml/1 tbsp tomato purée (paste)

15 ml/1 tbsp caster (superfine) sugar

Salt and freshly ground black pepper

150 ml/¼ pt/⅔ cup Soya Dream (see page 12)

50 g/2 oz/½ cup cooked rice

1 Fry (sauté) the onion, carrots and celery in the spread for 3 minutes, stirring, until softened but not browned.

2 Stir in the flour and cook for 1 minute.

3 Blend in the stock and add all the remaining ingredients except the Soya Dream and rice. Bring to the boil, reduce the heat and simmer for 45 minutes.

4 Purée the soup in a blender or food processor, then pass through a sieve (strainer) and pour back into the saucepan.

5 Stir in the Soya Dream and rice and heat through but do not boil. Taste and re-season, if necessary. Ladle into warm bowls and serve hot.

Carrot and Cumin Soup

40 g/1½ oz/3 tbsp soya spread

450 g/1 lb carrots, sliced

2 potatoes, chopped

1 onion, chopped

2.5 ml/½ tsp ground cumin

600 ml/1 pt/2½ cups lactose-free chicken stock

1 bay leaf

A pinch of cayenne

Salt and freshly ground black pepper

150 ml/¼ pt/⅔ cup soya milk

2 slices of dairy-free bread, cubed

1 garlic clove, halved

30 ml/2 tbsp sunflower oil

1   Heat 25 g/1 oz/2 tbsp of the spread in a saucepan and fry (sauté) the carrots, potatoes and onion for 2 minutes, stirring. Stir in the cumin and cook for 1 minute.

2   Add the stock, bay leaf, cayenne and a little salt and pepper. Bring to the boil, reduce the heat and simmer for 20 minutes. Discard the bay leaf.

3   Purée in a blender or food processor and return to the saucepan. Stir in the milk, taste and re-season, if necessary.

4   Add the garlic to the remaining spread and the oil, and fry the bread cubes, tossing until golden. Drain on kitchen paper (paper towels) and discard the garlic.

5   Ladle the soup into bowls and top with the croûtons.

Mighty Minestrone

Peperami is one of the few processed meats that do not contain lactose. However, it is always advisable to check the label.

SERVES 4–6

15 g/½ oz/1 tbsp soya spread

1 large onion, halved and thinly sliced

2 carrots, chopped

1 turnip, chopped

400 g/14 oz/1 large can of chopped tomatoes

1 bay leaf

2 lactose-free chicken or vegetable stock cubes

1 peperami stick, chopped (optional)

50 g/2 oz short-cut macaroni

425 g/15 oz/1 large can of haricot (navy) beans, drained

¼ small green cabbage, shredded

Salt and freshly ground black pepper

1 Heat the spread in a large saucepan and fry (sauté) the onion, carrots and turnip for 3 minutes, stirring.

2 Stir in the tomatoes. Fill the can with water and add to the pan. Repeat with a second canful of water.

3 Add the bay leaf and stock cubes, bring to the boil, reduce the heat and simmer gently for 30 minutes.

4 Discard the bay leaf and add all the remaining ingredients. Bring back to the boil, reduce the heat and simmer for a further 10–15 minutes until everything is really tender. Taste and re-season, if necessary.

Green Pea and Bacon Soup

SERVES 4

4 rashers (slices) of unsmoked streaky bacon, rinded and chopped

1 small onion, chopped

15 g/½ oz/1 tbsp soya spread

350 g/12 oz frozen peas

600 ml/1 pt/2½ cups lactose-free chicken or ham stock

Salt and freshly ground black pepper

15 ml/1 tbsp plain (all-purpose) flour

75 ml/5 tbsp soya milk

A pinch of grated nutmeg

1 Put half the bacon in a saucepan with the onion and soya spread. Fry (sauté) for 3 minutes, stirring until softened but not browned.

2 Add the peas, stock and a little salt and pepper. Bring to the boil, reduce the heat, part-cover and simmer gently for 10 minutes.

3 Purée in a blender or food processor.

4 Meanwhile, dry-fry the remaining bacon in the saucepan until crisp. Drain on kitchen paper (paper towels).

5 Blend the flour into the fat in the saucepan, then gradually blend in the soya milk until smooth. Return the purée to the pan, bring to the boil and simmer for 2 minutes, stirring. Taste, add the nutmeg and re-season, if necessary.

6 Ladle into warm bowls and sprinkle with the crisp bacon.

Chicken and Corn Chowder

1 chicken portion, all skin removed

450 ml/¾ pt/2 cups water

1 bunch of spring onions (scallions), chopped

2 potatoes, finely diced

Salt and freshly ground black pepper

320 g/12 oz/1 large can of sweetcorn (corn)

300 ml/½ pt/1¼ cups soya milk

30 ml/2 tbsp chopped fresh parsley

1 Put the chicken portion in a pan with the water. Bring to the boil, reduce the heat, part-cover and simmer gently for 45 minutes.

2 Carefully lift out the chicken, remove all meat from the bones, chop and reserve.

3 Add the spring onions, potatoes and some salt and pepper to the chicken stock and simmer for 10 minutes. Add the chicken and corn and stir in the milk.

4 Bring to the boil and cook for 2 minutes, stirring all the time.

5 Stir in the parsley and add more seasoning, if liked. Ladle into bowls and serve hot.

Aubergine and Red Pepper Soup with Rouille

SERVES 6

2 aubergines (eggplants)

2 red (bell) peppers

1 red onion, chopped

2 garlic cloves, crushed

2 tomatoes, skinned, seeded and chopped

90 ml/6 tbsp olive oil

90 ml/6 tbsp sunflower oil

600 ml/1 pt/2½ cups lactose-free chicken stock

Salt and freshly ground black pepper

1 red chilli, seeded and chopped

1 slice of dairy-free white bread, crusts removed

1 egg yolk

1 Grill (broil) the aubergines and peppers for about 20 minutes, turning until the skins are blackened. Place the peppers in a plastic bag.

2 Hold the aubergines under cold running water and peel off the skins. Chop the flesh and place in a saucepan.

3 Remove the skins from the peppers. Chop one and add to the aubergines with the onion, one of the garlic cloves, the tomatoes and 30 ml/2 tbsp each of the olive and sunflower oils.

4 Cook over a moderate heat, stirring occasionally, for 5 minutes until sizzling. Cover, reduce the heat and cook for a further 15 minutes, stirring occasionally.

5   Add the stock, bring to the boil, cover, reduce the heat and simmer for a further 10 minutes. Purée in a blender or food processor and return to the pan. Taste and re-season, if necessary.

6   Meanwhile, make the rouille. Put the chilli, the remaining red pepper and garlic, the bread and egg yolk in a blender. Add a sprinkling of salt and pepper. Run the machine until smooth, stopping and scraping down the sides as necessary.

7   With the machine running, add the remaining oils in a thin trickle until the mixture is thick and glossy, like mayonnaise. Taste and re-season, if necessary. Turn into a small bowl, cover in clingfilm (plastic wrap) and chill until required.

8   Ladle the soup into warm bowls, add a spoonful of the rouille to each and serve.

Lentil and Tomato Soup with Cardamom

SERVES 4

1 onion, chopped

10 ml/2 tsp olive oil

100 g/4 oz/⅔ cup red lentils

600 ml/1 pt/2½ cups tomato juice

300 ml/½ pt/1¼ cups lactose-free chicken or vegetable stock

15 ml/1 tbsp tomato purée (paste)

3 cardamom pods, split

Salt and freshly ground black pepper

20 ml/4 tsp soya yoghurt and 15 ml/1 tbsp chopped fresh coriander (cilantro), to garnish

1 Fry (sauté) the onion in the oil in a saucepan for 2 minutes, stirring, until softened but not browned.

2 Add all the remaining ingredients. Bring to the boil, reduce the heat and simmer gently for about 30 minutes until the lentils are completely soft. Discard the cardamom pods.

3 Taste and re-season, if necessary. Ladle into warm bowls and garnish each with a little yoghurt and a sprinkling of chopped coriander.

Velvet Leek and Potato Soup

25 g/1 oz/2 tbsp soya spread

1 onion, chopped

2 leeks, chopped

1 large potato, diced

600 ml/1 pt/2½ cups lactose-free chicken stock

Salt and white pepper

150 ml/¼ pt/⅔ cup soya milk

15 ml/1 tbsp chopped fresh parsley, to garnish

1 Heat the spread in a saucepan and fry (sauté) the onion, leeks and potato for 3 minutes, stirring, until softened but not browned.

2 Add the stock, then bring to the boil, reduce the heat, part-cover and simmer gently for about 30 minutes or until really tender.

3 Purée in a blender or food processor and return to the saucepan. Stir in the milk and season to taste.

4 Reheat, ladle into bowls and sprinkle with chopped parsley.

Pale Green Dream

Most mustards are safe, but do check the label.

1 ogen melon (or other melon with green flesh)

½ cucumber, peeled and sliced

2 ripe avocados

15 ml/1 tbsp lemon juice

45 ml/3 tbsp olive oil

45 ml/3 tbsp sunflower oil

30 ml/2 tbsp white wine vinegar

30 ml/2 tbsp apple juice

2.5 ml/½ tsp Dijon mustard

15 ml/1 tbsp chopped fresh parsley

15 ml/1 tbsp snipped fresh chives

Salt and freshly ground black pepper

Sprigs of watercress, to garnish

1 Halve the melon, discard the seeds, then scoop out the flesh using a melon baller or cut it into dice.

2 Halve the avocados, discard the stones (pits) and the rind and cut the flesh into neat slices. Toss in the lemon juice to prevent browning.

3 Arrange the melon balls or cubes in a small pile the centre of six individual plates. Surround with a ring of cucumber slices, then slices of avocado in a starburst pattern.

4 Whisk all the remaining ingredients together and drizzle over the salads. Garnish with sprigs of watercress and serve.

Spiced Banana and Corn Toppers

SERVES 4

5 eggs

2 bananas, thickly sliced

50 g/2 oz/1 cup fresh dairy-free white breadcrumbs

1.5 ml/¼ tsp chilli powder

5 ml/1 tsp sweet pimenton or paprika

Sunflower oil

200 g/7 oz/1 small can of sweetcorn (corn) with (bell) peppers

30 ml/2 tbsp dairy-free mayonnaise

4 slices of dairy-free granary bread, toasted

4 red or green pepper rings, to garnish

1 Beat one of the eggs. Add the bananas and toss to coat. Mix the breadcrumbs with the spices and use to coat the banana pieces.

2 Heat a little sunflower oil in a frying pan (skillet) and fry (sauté) the bananas, turning occasionally until golden. Drain on kitchen paper (paper towels) and keep warm.

3 Heat the sweetcorn in a saucepan and stir in the mayonnaise.

4 Meanwhile, fry the remaining eggs in a little more oil until cooked to your liking.

5 Put a slice of toast on each of four individual plates. Top with the sweetcorn, bananas and the eggs, and garnish each with a pepper ring. Serve hot.

Bruschetta

Ciabatta should not contain lactose or dairy products, but do check.

SERVES 4

4 canned anchovy fillets

45 ml/3 tbsp soya milk

1 garlic clove, halved

15 ml/1 tbsp pine nuts

5 ml/1 tsp lemon juice

45 ml/3 tbsp olive oil

4 thick slices of ciabatta bread, cut diagonally

4 ripe tomatoes, sliced

Freshly ground black pepper

8 fresh basil leaves, torn, to garnish

1 Soak the anchovies in the milk for 15 minutes. Drain.

2 With the machine running, drop them in a blender or food processor with the garlic, pine nuts and lemon juice. Stop and scrape down the sides. Run the machine again and trickle in 30 ml/2 tbsp of the olive oil to form a paste.

3 Brush one side of each of the bread slices with the remaining oil. Grill (broil) the oiled side until crisp and browned.

4 Turn the bread over and spread with the paste. Top with the sliced tomatoes and a good grinding of pepper. Grill again until the tomatoes are soft and the paste is bubbling.

5 Scatter the basil over and serve.

Crostini with Olives and Mushrooms

SERVES 4

8 slices of dairy-free French bread, cut diagonally

1 large garlic clove, halved

175 g/6 oz chestnut mushrooms, finely chopped

30 ml/2 tbsp olive oil

15 ml/1 tbsp dry vermouth

Freshly ground black pepper

50 g/2 oz stoned (pitted) black olives

5 ml/1 tsp lemon juice

15 ml/1 tbsp chopped fresh basil

1 Put the slices of bread on a baking (cookie) sheet and rub with the cut sides of the garlic clove. Reserve the garlic.

2 Bake the bread in a preheated oven at 180°C/350°F/gas mark 4 for 20 minutes until crisp and golden.

3 Crush the garlic and put in a saucepan with the mushrooms, half the oil, the vermouth and a good grinding of pepper. Cook gently, stirring for 5 minutes.

4 Meanwhile, put the olives and lemon juice in a blender or food processor and chop as finely as possible, stopping and scraping down the sides of the machine as necessary until a rough paste is formed.

5 Spread the olive paste on the bread and top with the mushrooms. Sprinkle with the basil and serve straight away.

Aubergine Dip with Crudités

1 large aubergine (eggplant)

1 spring onion (scallion), very finely chopped

1 small garlic clove, crushed

2 large ripe tomatoes, skinned, seeded and chopped

45 ml/3 tbsp olive oil

Lemon juice, to taste

Salt and freshly ground black pepper

15 ml/1 tbsp chopped fresh parsley

For the crudités:

2 carrots, cut into matchsticks

¼ cucumber, cut into matchsticks

1 red (bell) pepper, cut into thin strips

16 tiny button mushrooms

1 Grill (broil) the aubergine, turning occasionally, until the skin blackens and the flesh feels soft when squeezed.

2 When cool enough to handle, peel off the skin and discard, then chop the flesh finely and place in a bowl.

3 Add the spring onion, garlic and tomatoes and mix well.

4 Add the oil a drop or two at a time, beating well after each addition until the mixture is glistening but still quite thick. Add lemon juice and salt and pepper to taste.

5 Spoon into small pots and sprinkle with parsley. Arrange the crudités around and serve very cold.

Grilled Marinated Tofu on Toast

Marinate the tofu in advance for a very quick, easy snack.
Don't forget to check the label of the mustard.

SERVES 4

283 g/10½ oz/1 block of firm tofu

30 ml/2 tbsp soy sauce

45 ml/3 tbsp medium sherry

15 ml/1 tbsp dark brown sugar

5 ml/1 tsp ground ginger

15 ml/1 tbsp sunflower oil, plus extra for brushing

½ garlic clove, crushed

1.5 ml/¼ tsp made English mustard

4 small slices of dairy-free wholemeal bread

A little soya spread

1 Drain the tofu thoroughly in a sieve (strainer) over a bowl, then pat dry with kitchen paper (paper towels).

2 Whisk together all the remaining ingredients except the bread, soya spread and oil, until smooth.

3 Cut the tofu into four slices and place in a single layer in the marinade. Turn over. Chill, preferably overnight, turning occasionally until well soaked in the mixture.

4 Toast the bread under the grill (broiler). Spread with the soya spread. Place slabs of the tofu on top and brush with oil.

5 Grill (broil) for about 2 minutes or until bubbling. Serve immediately.

Sardine Pâté Crispers

SERVES 4

125 g/4½ oz/1 small can of sardines in oil, drained

40 g/1½ oz/3 tbsp soya spread

75 ml/5 tbsp soya yoghurt

2.5 ml/½ lemon juice

A few drops of Tabasco sauce

Salt and feshly ground black pepper

1 small onion, thinly sliced and separated into rings

15 ml/1 tbsp chopped fresh parsley

8 rye crispbreads, to serve

1 Put all the ingredients, except the onion and parsley, in a blender or food processor and run the machine until smooth.

2 Spread thickly on the crispbreads and top with the onion rings and parsley.

Peanut Rarebit

Try putting slices of tomato or cucumber or chopped celery or even a spoonful of sweet pickle on the toast before adding the topping.

SERVES 1

15 g/½ oz/1 tbsp smooth peanut butter

15 g/½ oz/1 tbsp soya spread

1 slice of dairy-free bread

A pinch of onion or garlic salt

1 Mash the peanut butter and soya spread thoroughly together.

2 Toast the bread on both sides.

3 Spread one side thickly with the peanut mixture and sprinkle with the onion or garlic salt.

4 Grill (broil) until bubbling and turning golden.

Pilchard Pots

This also makes a delicious sandwich filling, with slices of tomato and cucumber or some shredded lettuce.

SERVES 4

---

425 g/15 oz/1 large can of pilchards in tomato sauce

30 ml/2 tbsp dairy-free mayonnaise

15 ml/1 tbsp tomato purée (paste)

90 ml/6 tbsp soya yoghurt

5 ml/1 tsp red wine vinegar

1.5 ml/¼ tsp cayenne

15 ml/1 tbsp snipped fresh chives, to garnish

Toast, to serve

1 Empty the pilchards (including the bones) into a bowl and mash thoroughly.

2 Add all the remaining ingredients and beat well.

3 Turn into ramekin dishes (custard cups) and chill until ready to serve, if time allows.

4 Sprinkle with snipped chives and serve with toast.

Tofu Cakes

150 g/5 oz firm tofu, drained and finely chopped

1 large potato, finely grated

1 small onion, grated

30 ml/2 tbsp chopped fresh parsley

*30 ml/2 tbsp sunflower oil, plus extra for frying
(sautéing)*

Salt and freshly ground black pepper

75 g/3 oz/¾ cup self-raising (self-rising) wholemeal flour

150 ml/¼ pt/⅔ cup soya milk

Sweet pickle or tomato ketchup (catsup), to serve

1 Mix all the ingredients except the milk in a bowl.

2 Gradually beat in the milk to form a batter.

3 Heat a little oil in a large, heavy-based frying pan (skillet) and drop in spoonfuls of the batter.

4 Fry until cooked through and golden brown on both sides. Drain on kitchen paper (paper towels). Keep warm while cooking the remainder.

5 Serve hot with sweet pickle or tomato ketchup.

FISH AND VEGETABLE MAIN COURSES

You can eat all kinds of plain grilled (broiled), fried (sautéed) or baked fish without any qualms. And of course you can (and should) devour as many fresh vegetables as you can, every single day. So, for this section, I have developed some more unusual fish and veggie main courses for you to enjoy that will also impress your friends and family.

Monkfish Tabbouleh

For a vegetarian version, omit the fish and sprinkle with a handful of cashew nuts.

SERVES 4

---

225 g/8 oz/2 cups bulgar (cracked wheat)

600 ml/1 pt/2½ cups boiling water

350 g/12 oz monkfish, cut into large cubes

Salt and freshly ground black pepper

1 bunch of spring onions (scallions), trimmed, reserving the trimmings, and finely chopped

60 ml/4 tbsp chopped fresh parsley

30 ml/2 tbsp chopped fresh coriander (cilantro)

30 ml/2 tbsp chopped fresh mint

60 ml/4 tbsp olive oil

Finely grated rind and juice of ½ lemon

30 ml/2 tbsp white wine vinegar

1 garlic clove, crushed

5 cm/2 in piece of cucumber, chopped

100 g/4 oz cherry tomatoes, halved

1 Put the bulgar in a large bowl. Add the boiling water, stir and leave to stand for 30 minutes or until swollen, soft and the water has been absorbed. Drain and leave to cool.

2 Put the monkfish in a saucepan. Cover with water, add a little salt and pepper and the spring onion trimmings. Bring to the boil, reduce the heat, cover and simmer gently for 5 minutes until just tender. Drain and leave to cool. Discard the onion trimmings.

3 Tip the bulgar into a large salad bowl. Add all the remaining ingredients except the fish and toss well. Add the fish and gently toss in the salad. Season to taste.

4 Cover and chill for at least 2 hours before serving.

Trout with Cashew Nuts

SERVES 4

4 trout, cleaned and heads removed, if preferred

Salt and freshly ground black pepper

75 g/3 oz/⅓ cup soya spread

50 g/2 oz/½ cup raw cashew nuts

15 ml/1 tbsp lemon juice

30 ml/2 tbsp chopped fresh parsley

New potatoes and French (green) beans, to serve

1 Wipe the fish inside and out with kitchen paper (paper towels). Make several slashes on each side. Season with salt and pepper.

2 Heat the spread in a large frying pan (skillet). Add the fish and fry (sauté) for 3–4 minutes until golden brown underneath.

3 Turn over and add the nuts. Fry for a further 3 minutes until golden and cooked through.

4 Carefully transfer to warm plates, leaving the nuts in the pan.

5 Add the lemon juice and parsley to the pan with a little more salt and pepper. Heat through, stirring. Spoon the nut mixture over the fish and serve hot with new potatoes and French beans.

Smoked Mackerel and Potato Bowls

Make sure you use horseradish sauce, not creamed horseradish, which has dairy products in it. Alternatively, use grated fresh horseradish.

SERVES 4

---

450 g/1 lb baby new potatoes, scrubbed and halved

A sprig of fresh mint

4 ready-to-eat smoked mackerel fillets, skinned and cut into bite-sized pieces

100 g/4 oz fresh shelled or cooked frozen peas

45 ml/3 tbsp dairy-free mayonnaise

30 ml/2 tbsp sunflower oil

15 ml/1 tbsp lemon juice

10 ml/2 tsp horseradish sauce

Salt and freshly ground black pepper

Lettuce leaves

12 cherry tomatoes, halved, to garnish

1 Boil the potatoes in lightly salted water to which the mint has been added until just tender. Drain and tip into a large bowl, discarding the mint.

2 Add the fish and peas and mix gently.

3 Whisk together the mayonnaise, oil, lemon juice, horseradish sauce and a little salt and pepper and add to the bowl. Toss gently, but thoroughly.

4 Line four large soup bowls with lettuce leaves and spoon in the potato and fish mixture. Scatter the cherry tomatoes on top and serve.

Crab and Cucumber Gougère

2 quantities of Choux Pastry (see page 170)

25 g/1 oz/2 tbsp soya spread

300 ml/½ pt/1¼ cups soya milk

25 g/1 oz/¼ cup plain (all-purpose) flour

1 bouquet garni sachet

½ cucumber, finely chopped

170 g/6 oz/1 small can of white crabmeat, drained

5 ml/1 tsp anchovy essence (extract)

15 ml/1 tbsp chopped fresh dill (dill weed)

Freshly ground black pepper

Lemon juice, to taste

A tomato, avocado and onion salad, to serve

1 Prepare the pastry (paste).

2 Use a little spread to grease a 1.5 litre/2½ pt/6 cup shallow, ovenproof dish. Spoon the pastry all round the edge.

3 Blend the flour with a little of the milk in a saucepan. Stir in the remaining milk and soya spread and add the bouquet garni. Bring to the boil and cook, stirring, for 2 minutes. Discard the bouquet garni.

4 Squeeze the chopped cucumber to extract excess moisture. Stir into the sauce with the crabmeat, anchovy essence and dill. Season and sharpen with lemon juice to taste.

5 Spoon into the centre of the pastry ring. Bake in a preheated oven at 200°C/400°F/gas mark 6 for 40 minutes until the pastry is crisp, risen and golden. Serve hot with a tomato, avocado and onion salad.

Tandoori Fish with Tomato and Mango Rice

SERVES 4

450 g/1 lb any white fish fillet, skinned and bones removed

150 ml/¼ pt/⅔ cup soya yoghurt

15 ml/1 tbsp lemon juice

5 ml/1 tsp ground cumin

5 ml/1 tsp ground coriander (cilantro)

2.5 ml/½ tsp chilli powder

2.5 ml/½ tsp ground turmeric

Salt

175 g/6 oz/¾ cup basmati rice, rinsed

400 g/14 oz/1 large can of chopped tomatoes

300 ml/½ pt/1¼ cups water

1 fresh ripe mango

15 ml/1 tbsp chopped fresh coriander

Cucumber, tomatoes and salad leaves, to garnish

Poppadoms, to serve

1 Cut the fish into four equal pieces. Place in a shallow, ovenproof dish, in a single layer.

2 Mix the yoghurt, lemon juice, spices and a good pinch of salt together and pour over the fish. Turn the fillets to coat completely, cover and leave to marinate for 2 hours.

3 Place the fish in a preheated oven at 180°C/350°F/gas mark 4 for 20 minutes, basting occasionally.

4 As soon as you put the fish in the oven to cook, put the rice in a saucepan with the tomatoes and water. Bring to the boil, reduce the heat, cover and cook gently for 20 minutes until the rice is tender and has absorbed the liquid.

5 Meanwhile, peel the mango, cut all the flesh off the stone (pit) and cut into neat pieces.

6 When the rice is cooked, stir in the coriander and mango and season to taste.

7 Spoon the rice on to warm plates and top with the fish. Garnish with cucumber, tomatoes and salad leaves and serve with poppadoms.

Grilled Salmon with
Watercress Hollandaise

SERVES 4

1 bunch of watercress

4 salmon tail fillets, about 175 g/6 oz each

Salt and freshly ground black pepper

2 eggs

30 ml/2 tbsp lemon juice

100 g/4 oz/½ cup soya spread, melted

30 ml/2 tbsp chopped fresh parsley

New potatoes and mangetout (snow peas), to serve

1 Trim the feathery stalks off the watercress. Choose four sprigs for garnish and chop the remainder.

2 Put the salmon on the grill (broiler) rack and season lightly. Grill (broil) for about 5–6 minutes until just cooked through. Do not overcook.

3 Meanwhile, whisk the eggs in a saucepan with the lemon juice.

4 Place over a gentle heat and gradually whisk in the melted soya spread, whisking all the time until thick and creamy. Do not allow to boil.

5 Remove from the heat and stir in the watercress, parsley and salt and pepper to taste.

6 Transfer the fish to warm plates. Spoon a little of the sauce over and garnish with the reserved watercress sprigs. Serve with new potatoes and mangetout.

Salmon in Filo Pastry

425 g/15 oz/1 large can of pink or red salmon, drained

4 large sheets of filo pastry (paste)

40 g/1½ oz/3 tbsp soya spread, melted

4 cup mushrooms, sliced

1 large tomato, chopped

5 ml/1 tsp dried oregano

Freshly ground black pepper

120 ml/4 fl oz/½ cup passata (sieved tomatoes)

New potatoes and French (green) beans, to serve

1 Remove the skin from the salmon and divide the fish into four equal amounts but, preferably, leave in the bones.

2 Put a sheet of filo pastry on a board and brush with a little of the melted soya spread. Fold in half to form a square and brush again.

3 Top with a quarter of the mushroom slices and chopped tomato and sprinkle with some of the oregano. Add a portion of salmon. Season with pepper.

4 Draw the pastry up over the fish, pinching it together to form a pouch. Place on a baking (cookie) sheet, lightly brushed with a little of the soya spread.

5 Repeat with the remaining pastry and filling.

6 Bake in a preheated oven at 190°C/375°F/gas mark 5 for about 15 minutes until golden brown.

7 Meanwhile, heat the passata in a small saucepan.

8 Transfer one parcel to each of four warm plates. Spoon a little passata around and serve with new potatoes and French beans.

Spicy Prawn Fajitas

SERVES 4

1 red onion, chopped

1 large garlic clove, crushed

100 g/4 oz button mushrooms, sliced

30 ml/2 tbsp olive oil

1 red chilli, seeded and chopped

400 g/14 oz/1 large can of chopped tomatoes

30 ml/2 tbsp tomato purée (paste)

5 ml/1 tsp caster (superfine) sugar

Salt and freshly ground black pepper

225 g/8 oz uncooked peeled tiger prawns (jumbo shrimp), thawed if frozen

A few drops of Tabasco sauce (optional)

8 large flour tortillas

¼ iceberg lettuce, finely shredded

5 cm/2 in piece of cucumber, finely chopped

1 small red (bell) pepper, finely chopped

90 ml/6 tbsp soya yoghurt

1 Fry (sauté) the onion, garlic and mushrooms in the oil for 3 minutes, stirring until softened but not browned.

2 Add the chilli, tomatoes, tomato purée, sugar and a little salt and pepper. Bring to the boil and boil fairly rapidly for about 5 minutes, stirring occasionally, until really thick and pulpy.

3 Add the prawns and continue to bubble until the prawns are pink. Taste and re-season, adding a few drops of Tabasco, if liked.

4 Meanwhile, warm the tortillas according to the packet directions.

5 Divide the lettuce, cucumber and pepper between the tortillas. Top with the prawns and spoon a little yoghurt over the top. Roll up and serve.

Pissaladière

SERVES 4

175 g/6 oz/1½ cups plain (all-purpose) flour

5 ml/1 tsp baking powder

5 ml/1 tsp ground cinnamon

Salt

75 g/3 oz/⅓ cup soya spread

3 onions, sliced

1 garlic clove, crushed

30 ml/2 tbsp olive oil

450 g/1 lb tomatoes, roughly chopped

15 ml/1 tbsp tomato purée (paste)

2.5 ml/½ tsp caster (superfine) sugar

Freshly ground black pepper

50 g/2 oz/1 small can of anchovy fillets, drained

6 black olives

6 green olives

15 ml/1 tbsp chopped fresh parsley

1 Mix the flour, baking powder, cinnamon and a pinch of salt in a bowl.

2 Add the soya spread and rub in with your fingertips until the mixture is almost forming a dough.

3 Mix with cold water, a teaspoonful at a time, until a soft but not sticky dough is formed.

4 Roll out on a lightly floured surface and use to line a 20 cm/8 in flan tin (pie pan). Prick the base with a fork and line with crumpled foil.

5 Bake in a preheated oven at 200°C/400°F/gas mark 6 for 10 minutes. Remove the foil and return to the oven for 5 minutes to dry out.

6 Meanwhile, cook the onions and garlic in the oil, in a large pan, for 3 minutes until softened. Add the tomatoes, tomato purée, sugar and a little salt and pepper and simmer for 8 minutes until pulpy.

7 Turn into the pastry case (pie shell) and decorate with the anchovies and olives.

8 Return to the oven for 10 minutes. Sprinkle with parsley and serve.

Savoury Egg Pasta

For a delicious variation, use a drained 185 g/6½ oz/small can of tuna instead of the eggs.

SERVES 4

225 g/8 oz pasta shapes

1 large onion, finely chopped

1 garlic clove, crushed

75 g/3 oz/⅓ cup soya spread

225 g/8 oz spring (collard) greens, shredded

400 g/14 oz/1 large can of chopped tomatoes

5 ml/1 tsp caster (superfine) sugar

A good pinch of dried basil

Salt and freshly ground black pepper

3 hard-boiled (hard-cooked) eggs, roughly chopped

30 ml/2 tbsp plain (all-purpose) flour

300 ml/½ pt/1¼ cups soya milk

1 large bay leaf

50 g/2 oz/1 cup fresh dairy-free white breadcrumbs

1 Cook the pasta according to the packet directions until just tender. Drain.

2 Cook the onion and garlic in 40 g/1½ oz/3 tbsp of the spread for 2 minutes, stirring.

3 Add the greens, tomatoes, sugar, basil and a little salt and pepper. Cover and simmer for 5 minutes, stirring occasionally.

4 Use a little of the remaining spread to grease a 1.2 litre/2 pt/5 cup ovenproof dish.

5 Spoon half the pasta into the dish. Cover with a layer of the eggs, then add the remaining pasta.

6 Blend the flour with a little of the soya milk in a saucepan. Blend in the remaining milk and add 15 g/ ½ oz/1 tbsp of the remaining spread and the bay leaf. Bring to the boil and simmer for 2 minutes, stirring all the time. Season to taste and discard the bay leaf.

7 Pour over the pasta. Sprinkle with the breadcrumbs and dot with the remaining spread. Bake in a preheated oven at 190°C/375°F/gas mark 5 for about 20 minutes until hot through and turning golden on top.

Spicy Lentil and Chestnut Mushroom Rissoles

SERVES 4

225 g/8 oz/1⅓ cups brown lentils, soaked for 2 hours in cold water

1 onion, finely chopped

100 g/4 oz chestnut mushrooms, finely chopped

50 g/2 oz/¼ cup soya spread

30 ml/2 tbsp chopped fresh coriander (cilantro)

1 fresh green chilli, seeded and chopped

5 ml/1 tsp ground cumin

Salt and freshly ground black pepper

75 g/3 oz/1½ cups fresh dairy-free wholemeal breadcrumbs

1 egg, beaten

Flour, for dusting

90 ml/6 tbsp sunflower oil, for frying (sautéing)

300 ml/½ pt/1¼ cups passata (sieved tomatoes)

5 ml/1 tsp caster (superfine) sugar

30 ml/2 tbsp soya yoghurt

Brown rice and a green salad, to serve

---

1 Drain the soaked lentils and place in a saucepan. Cover with water. Bring to the boil and boil rapidly for 10 minutes, reduce the heat, cover and simmer gently for about 1 hour or until the lentils are really soft and all the liquid has been absorbed.

2 Meanwhile, fry (sauté) the onion and mushrooms in the soya spread for 2 minutes, stirring.

3 Stir in half the coriander, the chilli, cumin and a little salt and pepper to taste.

4 Blend in the breadcrumbs and mix with the beaten egg to bind. Dust your hands with flour and shape the mixture into 16 cakes.

5 Heat the sunflower oil in a large frying pan (skillet) and fry the rissoles in two batches until golden brown on each side. Drain on kitchen paper (paper towels).

6 Meanwhile, heat the passata with the remaining coriander, the sugar and salt and pepper to taste.

7 Arrange the rissoles on four warm plates. Spoon the sauce over and add a swirl of yoghurt. Serve with brown rice and a green salad.

Spinach and Sweetcorn Roulade

SERVES 4

350 g/12 oz spinach, well washed and torn into pieces

25 g/1 oz/2 tbsp soya spread

A good pinch of grated nutmeg

4 eggs, separated

Salt and freshly ground black pepper

2 spring onions (scallions), finely chopped

30 ml/2 tbsp cornflour (cornstarch)

150 ml/¼ pt/⅔ cup soya milk

1 bay leaf

200 g/7 oz/1 small can of sweetcorn (corn)

190 g/6¾ oz/1 small can of pimientos, drained

225 g/8 oz/1 small can of tomatoes

A few drops of Tabasco sauce

New potatoes, to serve

1 Put the spinach in a saucepan with no extra water. Cover and cook for 5 minutes until tender. Drain off any liquid and chop finely with scissors.

2 Beat in half the soya spread, the nutmeg, egg yolks and a little salt and pepper.

3 Whisk the egg whites until stiff and fold into the spinach with a metal spoon.

4 Line an 18 × 28 cm/7 × 11 in Swiss roll tin (jelly roll pan) with non-stick baking parchment, so that it comes about 5 cm/2 in above the rim all round.

5   Turn the mixture into the tin and level the surface. Bake in a preheated oven at 200°C/400°F/gas mark 6 for about 20 minutes until risen, golden and just firm to the touch.

6   Meanwhile, fry (sauté) the spring onions in the remaining spread for 3 minutes until softened but not browned.

7   Remove from the heat and blend in the cornflour, then a little of the milk. Stir in the remaining milk and add the bay leaf.

8   Return to the heat, bring to the boil and cook for 2 minutes until thick and smooth. Stir in the sweetcorn and season to taste.

9   Purée the pimientos and tomatoes in a blender or food processor and add Tabasco, salt and pepper to taste. Heat through in a saucepan.

10 Turn the cooked roulade out on to a clean sheet of baking parchment. Remove the used baking paper. Spread with the sweetcorn mixture and roll up, using the paper as a guide.

11 Spoon a pool of the sauce on to four warm plates. Cut the roulade into slices and arrange on top. Serve with new potatoes.

Rice and Vegetable Stir-fry

SERVES 4

175 g/6 oz/¾ cup long-grain rice

45 ml/3 tbsp sunflower oil

4 spring onions (scallions), cut into short lengths

1 carrot, cut into thin matchsticks

5 cm/2 in piece of cucumber, cut into thin matchsticks

100 g/4 oz mangetout (snow peas)

100 g/4 oz baby sweetcorn (corn) cobs

1 red (bell) pepper, cut into thin strips

100 g/4 oz button mushrooms, sliced

2.5 cm/1 in piece of stem ginger in syrup, finely chopped

1 garlic clove, crushed

30 ml/2 tbsp soy sauce

1 Boil the rice in plenty of lightly salted water for 10 minutes or until just tender. Drain, rinse with boiling water and drain again.

2 Meanwhile, heat the oil in a wok or large frying pan (skillet). Add all the remaining ingredients except the soy sauce and stir-fry for 5 minutes.

3 Add the rice and toss until heated. Sprinkle in the soy sauce, toss again and serve.

Tagliatelle with Pesto and Oyster Mushrooms

SERVES 4

20 fresh basil leaves

1 large sprig of fresh parsley

100 g/4 oz/1 cup pine nuts

1 large garlic clove

1 canned anchovy fillet

90 ml/6 tbsp olive oil

Salt and freshly ground black pepper

350 g/12 oz tagliatelle

25 g/1 oz/2 tbsp soya spread

100 g/4 oz oyster mushrooms, sliced

1 onion, finely chopped

A mixed salad, to serve

1 Using a blender or food processor, with the machine running, drop in the basil and parsley, then the pine nuts, garlic and anchovy. Stop the machine and scrape down the sides as necessary.

2 Gradually trickle in the olive oil until a glistening paste is formed. Season to taste with salt and pepper.

3 Cook the tagliatelle according to the packet directions. Drain and return to the saucepan.

4 Meanwhile, melt the spread in a frying pan (skillet) and cook the mushrooms and onion for 3–4 minutes until soft and lightly golden.

5 Add the pesto and the onion mixture to the pasta and toss over a gentle heat until every strand is coated.

6 Pile on to warm plates and serve with a mixed salad.

Ratatouille with Chickpeas and Eggs

SERVES 4

1 onion, sliced

1 aubergine (eggplant), sliced

2 courgettes (zucchini), sliced

1 red (bell) pepper, cut into thin strips

1 green pepper, cut into thin strips

2 large tomatoes, cut into wedges

45 ml/3 tbsp olive oil

45 ml/3 tbsp red wine or water

30 ml/2 tbsp tomato purée (paste)

5 ml/1 tsp dried oregano

Salt and freshly ground black pepper

5 ml/1 tsp caster (superfine) sugar

*430 g/15½ oz/1 large can of chickpeas
(garbanzos), drained*

4 eggs

15 ml/1 tbsp chopped fresh parsley, to garnish

Crusty bread (see page 159), to serve

1 Put all the prepared vegetables in a large frying pan (skillet) with the oil. Cook for about 4 minutes, stirring, until softening.

2 Add the wine or water, tomato purée, oregano, some salt and pepper and the sugar. Stir well and bring to the boil. Cover with a lid or foil, reduce the heat and simmer gently for 15–20 minutes until everything is tender.

3 Stir in the chickpeas, then make four wells in the mixture.

4 Break an egg into each well, re-cover and cook for about 10 minutes, checking every few minutes until the eggs are cooked to your liking.

5 Sprinkle with parsley and serve straight from the pan with crusty bread.

Soya Bean Roast with Curried Rice Salad

SERVES 6

2 × 425 g/15 oz/large cans of soya beans, drained

50 g/2 oz/¼ cup soya spread, plus a little for greasing

45 ml/3 tbsp dried dairy-free breadcrumbs

1 large onion, finely chopped

1 carrot, grated

1 potato, grated

1 turnip, grated

30 ml/2 tbsp curry powder

50 g/2 oz/1 cup fresh dairy-free wholemeal breadcrumbs

45 ml/3 tbsp mango chutney

Salt and freshly ground black pepper

2 eggs, beaten

175 g/6 oz/¾ cup basmati rice, rinsed

45 ml/3 tbsp dairy-free mayonnaise

5 cm/2 in piece of cucumber, diced

2 tomatoes, chopped

30 ml/2 tbsp toasted flaked (slivered) almonds

1 Empty the soya beans into a bowl and mash with a potato masher.
2 Grease a 900 g/2 lb loaf tin (pan) with a little soya spread and dust with the dried breadcrumbs.

3 Melt the measured spread in a saucepan. Add the prepared vegetables and half the curry powder and fry (sauté), stirring, for 5 minutes.

4 Stir this mixture into the soya beans with the fresh wholemeal breadcrumbs and 30 ml/2 tbsp of the mango chutney. Season well.

5 Mix in the beaten eggs, then turn the mixture into the prepared tin and smooth the surface.

6 Cover with foil and bake in a preheated oven at 190°C/375°F/gas mark 5 for 1½ hours until firm to the touch. Cool for 10 minutes, then turn out on to a serving dish.

7 Meanwhile, cook the rice in plenty of boiling, lightly salted water for 10 minutes until tender. Drain, rinse with cold water and drain again.

8 Mix the remaining curry powder and mango chutney with the mayonnaise and a little seasoning. Stir in the rice, cucumber and tomatoes.

9 Slice the warm or cold loaf and serve with the curried rice, garnished with the almonds.

Smoked Tofu with Asparagus Stir-fry

15 ml/1 tbsp sunflower oil

15 ml/1 tbsp sesame oil

450 g/1 lb thin asparagus, trimmed and cut into short lengths

1 red (bell) pepper, cut into thin strips

225 g/8 oz smoked tofu, cubed

15 ml/1 tbsp light brown sugar

15 ml/1 tbsp white wine vinegar

15 ml/1 tbsp soy sauce

1.5 ml/¼ tsp cayenne

150 ml/¼ pt/⅔ cup lactose-free vegetable stock

10 ml/2 tsp sesame seeds

Plain rice, to serve

1 Heat the oils in a wok or large frying pan (skillet).

2 Add the asparagus and pepper and stir-fry for 5 minutes.

3 Add all the remaining ingredients, except the sesame seeds. Bring to the boil and cook for 7 minutes, stirring occasionally.

4 Sprinkle with the sesame seeds and serve straight away with plain rice.

MEAT AND POULTRY MAIN COURSES

You can, of course enjoy any meat or poultry cooked any way you like as long as it doesn't have a creamy sauce or a cheesy topping. But many commercially prepared meals do include hidden dairy products, so beware. Here I have created some versions of popular favourites that normally contain dairy products in some form or another, plus a selection of other recipes that are just too good to be left out.

Very Slow-cooked Braised Beef in Red Wine

Be sure that the brand of mustard you buy is safe for you.

SERVES 4

---

700 g/1½ lb braising steak, trimmed of fat and cubed

45 ml/3 tbsp plain (all-purpose) flour

Salt and freshly ground black pepper

45 ml/3 tbsp sunflower oil

1 large onion, thinly sliced

2 carrots, cut into small dice

300 ml/½ pt/1¼ cups red wine

450 ml/¾ pt/2 cups lactose-free beef stock

15 ml/1 tbsp brandy

15 ml/1 tbsp tomato purée (paste)

2.5 ml/½ tsp Dijon mustard

5 ml/1 tsp caster (superfine) sugar

1 bouquet garni sachet

175 g/6 oz whole button mushrooms

Jacket potatoes and broccoli, to serve

1 Toss the meat in the flour, seasoned with a little salt and pepper.

2 Heat 15 ml/1 tbsp of the oil in a flameproof casserole (Dutch oven) and fry (sauté) the onion and carrots for 2 minutes, stirring. Remove from the pan with a draining spoon.

3 Add the remaining oil and brown the meat on all sides. Remove from the pan.

4 Add any remaining flour to the pan, then blend in the wine, stock, brandy, tomato purée, mustard and sugar. Season well and return the carrots, onion and meat to the liquid. Bring to the boil and add the bouquet garni and mushrooms.

5 Cover and place in a preheated oven at 150°C/300°F/ gas mark 2 for 4 hours or until the meat is really tender and bathed in a rich sauce. Discard the bouquet garni, taste and re-season, if necessary.

6 Serve hot with jacket potatoes and broccoli.

Steak Strips Sizzle with Crunchy Noodles

SERVES 4

350 g/12 oz thin-cut beef steak, cut into narrow strips

15 ml/1 tbsp lemon juice

30 ml/2 tbsp sunflower oil

1 large onion, finely chopped

100 g/4 oz button mushrooms, sliced

175 g/6 oz fresh spinach, well washed and shredded

45 ml/3 tbsp Worcestershire sauce

30 ml/2 tbsp apple juice

30 ml/2 tbsp chopped fresh parsley

225 g/8 oz tagliatelle or other flat noodles

25 g/1 oz/2 tbsp soya spread

25 g/1 oz/½ cup fresh dairy-free white breadcrumbs

25 g/1 oz/¼ cup chopped nuts

1 Place the steak in a shallow dish and toss in the lemon juice. Leave to stand for at least 2 hours.

2 Heat the oil in a large frying pan (skillet) or wok. Add the onion and cook for 2 minutes, stirring, to soften. Add the steak and mushrooms and toss for 2 minutes. Add the spinach, Worcestershire sauce and apple juice. Cover with foil or a lid and cook for 3 minutes.

3 Meanwhile, boil the tagliatelle in lightly salted water for 10 minutes or until just tender, then drain. Melt the soya spread in the saucepan and add the breadcrumbs and nuts. Toss over a fairly high heat until golden, then return the noodles to the pan and toss to coat.

4 Pile the noodles on warm plates. Top with the steak mixture and serve.

Rich Weekday Mince with Baby Vegetables

SERVES 4

2 large onions, chopped

450 g/1 lb minced (ground) beef

30 ml/2 tbsp sunflower oil

45 ml/3 tbsp plain (all-purpose) flour

750 ml/1¼ pts/3 cups lactose-free beef stock

1 bay leaf

Salt and freshly ground black pepper

225 g/8 oz whole baby carrots, scraped

450 g/1 lb whole baby new potatoes, scrubbed

8 whole baby turnips, peeled

100 g/4 oz baby sweetcorn (corn) cobs

Crusty bread (see page 159), to serve

1 Fry (sauté) the onions and beef in the oil in a flameproof casserole (Dutch oven) for about 5 minutes, stirring, until the meat is no longer pink and all the grains are separate.

2 Stir in the flour and cook for 1 minute.

3 Blend in the stock and bring to the boil, stirring.

4 Add the bay leaf, seasoning and the vegetables. Cover and cook in a preheated oven at 160°C/325°F/gas mark 3 for 2 hours.

5 Discard the bay leaf, taste and re-season, if necessary. Ladle into warm soup bowls and serve with crusty bread.

Beef Stroganoff with Artichokes

SERVES 4

25 g/1 oz/2 tbsp soya spread

2 large onions, sliced

450 g/1 lb braising steak, cut into thin strips

450 ml/¾ pt/2 cups lactose-free beef stock

Salt and freshly ground black pepper

30 ml/2 tbsp plain (all-purpose) flour

30 ml/2 tbsp water

30 ml/2 tbsp tomato purée (paste)

150 ml/¼ pt/⅔ cup soya yoghurt

425 g/15 oz/1 large can of artichoke hearts, drained and quartered

Plain rice and a green salad, to serve

1 Heat the spread in a flameproof casserole (Dutch oven) and fry (sauté) the onions for 2 minutes, stirring.

2 Add the steak and fry for a further 2 minutes, stirring.

3 Add the stock and a little salt and pepper. Bring to the boil, cover, reduce the heat and simmer very gently for 1½ hours or until the beef is really tender.

4 Blend the flour with the water. Stir in a little of the hot beef liquid, then stir this into the casserole. Bring to the boil, stirring, and cook for 2 minutes.

5 Add the tomato purée, yoghurt and artichoke hearts. Reheat but do not boil. Taste and re-season, if necessary.

6 Serve with rice and a green salad.

Rich Lamb and Bean Hot-pot

SERVES 4

176 g/6 oz/1 cup flageolet beans, soaked overnight in cold water

450 ml/¾ pt/2 cups water

1 lactose-free lamb stock cube

30 ml/2 tbsp redcurrant jelly (clear conserve)

2 leeks, sliced

2 lambs' kidneys, cored and chopped

8 best end of neck lamb cutlets

Salt and freshly ground black pepper

15 ml/1 tbsp chopped fresh rosemary

700 g/1½ lb potatoes, scrubbed and sliced

15 g/½ oz/1 tbsp soya spread

Leaf spinach, to serve

1 Drain the beans and place in a saucepan with the water. Bring to the boil and boil rapidly for 10 minutes. Reduce the heat, part-cover and simmer gently for 1 hour. Stir in the stock and redcurrant jelly until dissolved. Turn into a shallow, 2.25 litre/4 pt/10 cup ovenproof dish.

2 Add the leeks, kidneys and cutlets and season with salt, pepper and the rosemary.

3 Layer the potatoes on the top. Dot with the soya spread and season again. Cover with foil and bake in a preheated oven at 160°C/325°F/gas mark 3 for 1½ hours.

4 Remove the foil and continue cooking for a further hour until everything is really tender and the top is turning golden. Serve with leaf spinach.

Moroccan Lamb

SERVES 4

700 g/1½ lb boned shoulder of lamb, trimmed of fat and diced

12 button (pearl) onions, peeled

1 large garlic clove, crushed

1 green chilli, seeded and chopped

1.5 ml/¼ tsp ground cinnamon

1.5 ml/¼ tsp ground ginger

Salt and freshly ground black pepper

900 ml/1½ pts/3¾ cups lactose-free lamb stock

10 ml/2 tsp tomato purée (paste)

225 g/8 oz/1⅓ cups couscous

100 g/4 oz/⅔ cup ready-to-eat dried apricots, halved

2 courgettes (zucchini), diced

2 carrots, diced

1 green (bell) pepper, diced

30 ml/2 tbsp chopped fresh coriander (cilantro)

30 ml/2 tbsp chopped fresh parsley

1 Put the lamb and onions in a large saucepan with the garlic, chilli, spices, a little salt and pepper, the lamb stock and tomato purée. Bring to the boil, stirring. Reduce the heat, cover and simmer gently for 1½ hours.

2 Meanwhile, put the couscous in a bowl and add just enough boiling water to cover. Leave to stand for 5 minutes. Tip into a steamer or sieve (strainer).

3 Add the apricots and vegetables to the lamb mixture with half the herbs, top with the steamer of couscous and cook for a further 15 minutes.

4 Fluff up the couscous with a fork. If necessary, boil the stew rapidly to reduce the liquid to a thick sauce. Taste and adjust the seasoning.

5 Spoon the couscous on to warm plates. Spoon the lamb mixture on top and sprinkle with the remaining herbs before serving.

Red Lamb with Rosemary

SERVES 4
350 g/12 oz lamb neck fillet, cut into 12 thin slices
40 g/1½ oz/3 tbsp soya spread
1 red onion, finely chopped
1 cooked beetroot (red beet), finely diced
30 ml/2 tbsp chopped fresh rosemary
1 garlic clove, crushed
15 ml/1 tbsp tomato purée (paste)
30 ml/2 tbsp redcurrant jelly (clear conserve)
150 ml/¼ pt/⅔ cup lactose-free lamb or chicken stock
10 ml/2 tsp red wine vinegar
15 ml/1 tbsp chopped fresh parsley, to garnish
Creamed potatoes and French (green) beans, to serve

1 Place the lamb slices one at a time in a plastic bag and beat with a rolling pin or meat mallet to flatten.

2 Fry (sauté) the lamb in 25 g/1 oz/2 tbsp of the spread for about 2 minutes on each side until golden brown and just cooked through. Remove and keep warm.

3 Melt the remaining spread in the pan and fry the onion for 2 minutes until softened slightly. Add all the remaining ingredients and stir until the jelly dissolves, then bring to the boil, reduce the heat and simmer until slightly thickened. Taste and re-season, if necessary.

4 Transfer the lamb to warm plates and pour any juices back into the sauce in the pan.

5 Spoon the sauce over the lamb and garnish with chopped parsley. Serve with creamed potatoes and French beans.

Bacon and Bean Quiche

1 quantity of Shortcrust Pastry (see page 168)

3 rashers (slices) of streaky bacon, rinded and cut into small pieces

400 g/14 oz/1 large can of baked beans

2 eggs

150 ml/¼ pt/⅔ cup soya milk

Salt and freshly ground black pepper

2.5 ml/½ tsp dried mixed herbs

15 ml/1 tbsp chopped fresh parsley

30 ml/2 tbsp crushed cornflakes

Pickles and a mixed salad, to serve

1   Make up the pastry (paste), roll out and use to line a 20 cm/8 in flan dish (pie pan), placed on a baking (cookie) sheet.

2   Prick the base with a fork, line with crumpled foil and bake in a preheated oven at 200°C/400°F/gas mark 6 for 10 minutes. Remove the foil and return to the oven for 5 minutes to dry out.

3   Dry-fry the bacon in a frying pan (skillet) until crisp. Scatter in the base of the flan and cover with the beans.

4   Beat the eggs, soya milk and some salt and pepper together with the mixed herbs and parsley and pour into the flan.

5   Bake in the oven at 190°C/375°F/gas mark 5 for 30 minutes. Sprinkle the crushed cornflakes over the top and return to the oven for a further 10–15 minutes until the filling is set. Serve warm or cold with pickles and a mixed salad.

Hot Sweet and Sour Ribs

SERVES 4

1 kg/2¼ lb Chinese pork spare ribs

1 onion, finely chopped

1 green (bell) pepper, chopped

1 red pepper, chopped

30 ml/2 tbsp sunflower oil

228 g/8 oz/1 small can of pineapple pieces in natural juice, drained, reserving the juice

15 ml/1 tbsp light brown sugar

30 ml/2 tbsp tomato ketchup (catsup)

10 ml/2 tsp soy sauce

15 ml/1 tbsp chilli relish

Salt and freshly ground black pepper

30 ml/2 tbsp red wine vinegar

15 ml/1 tbsp cornflour (cornstarch)

Rice and Vegetable Stir-fry (see page 80), to serve

1 Put the ribs in a roasting tin (pan) in a single layer. Roast in a preheated oven at 200°C/400°F/gas mark 6 for 10 minutes.

2 Meanwhile, fry (sauté) the onion and peppers in the oil for 2 minutes.

3 Make up the pineapple juice to 300 ml/½ pt/1¼ cups with water. Add to the pan.

4 Chop the pineapple and add, together with the sugar, ketchup, soy sauce, chilli relish and a little salt and pepper.

5 Bring to the boil and simmer for 1 minute. Blend the vinegar and cornflour together, stir in and cook for 1 further minute.

6 Spoon the sauce over the ribs and cook for 45 minutes, turning and basting occasionally, until stickily glazed and really tender.

7 Serve with Rice and Vegetable Stir-fry.

Sage and Onion Sausage Toad with Carrot Gravy

Choose good-quality sausages and check the label to make sure they do not contain any dairy products.

SERVES 4

---

1 quantity of Yorkshire Pudding batter (see page 172)

8 thick pork sausages

3 onions, finely chopped

30 ml/2 tbsp sunflower oil

15 ml/1 tbsp chopped fresh sage

15 g/½ oz/1 tbsp soya spread

2 large carrots, grated

1 potato, grated

450 ml/¾ pt/2 cups lactose-free vegetable or chicken stock

Salt and freshly ground black pepper

1 small bay leaf

Creamed potatoes and peas, to serve

1 Make up the batter.

2 Put the sausages in an 18 × 28 cm/7 × 11 in shallow baking tin (pan) with the oil and two of the onions.

3 Place towards the top of a preheated oven at 220°C/ 425°F/gas mark 7 for about 5 minutes until really sizzling.

4 Pour in the batter and sprinkle with the sage. Return to the oven and cook for about 35–40 minutes until risen, crisp and golden.

5 Meanwhile, melt the spread in a saucepan. Fry (sauté) the remaining onion, the carrots and potato for 3 minutes, stirring until lightly golden.

6 Add the stock, a little salt and pepper and the bay leaf. Bring back to the boil, reduce the heat and simmer gently for 10 minutes or until the vegetables are really soft. Discard the bay leaf.

7 Purée in a blender or food processor and return to the pan. Taste and re-season, if necessary.

8 Serve the toad with the carrot gravy, creamed potatoes and peas.

Baked Gammon with Potato Cake

Wholegrain mustard should not be a problem, but do check the label.

SERVES 4

---

50 g/2 oz/¼ cup soya spread

450 g/1 lb potatoes, scrubbed and very thinly sliced

1 garlic clove, crushed

30 ml/2 tbsp chopped fresh parsley

Salt and freshly ground black pepper

300 ml/½ pt/1¼ cups soya yoghurt

1 egg, beaten

50 g/2 oz/1 small can of anchovy fillets, drained

700 g/1½ lb gammon joint

300 ml/½ pt/1¼ cups medium cider

1 bay leaf

15 ml/1 tbsp wholegrain mustard

15 ml/1 tbsp clear honey

15 ml/1 tbsp cornflour (cornstarch)

15 ml/1 tbsp water

Broccoli, to serve

1 Grease a 1.2 litre/2 pt/5 cup ovenproof dish with a little of the spread.

2 Layer the potatoes, garlic, parsley and a little salt and pepper in the dish, dotting each layer with the spread.

3 Whisk the yoghurt and egg together and pour over the potatoes.

4   Arrange the anchovies in a criss-cross pattern over the top. Cover with foil.

5   Put the gammon in a pan of water and bring to the boil. Discard the water.

6   Place the gammon in a casserole dish (Dutch oven). Pour the cider around, add the bay leaf and cover.

7   Place the meat just below the centre and the potatoes towards the top of a preheated oven at 190°C/375°F/ gas mark 5 for 45 minutes.

8   Remove the foil and the casserole lid. Lift out the gammon and cut off any rind. Return to the casserole. Mix the mustard and honey together and spoon over the surface, then cook everything for a further 20 minutes until the potatoes and gammon are cooked through and browning on top.

9   Transfer the gammon to a carving dish. Blend the cornflour with the water and stir into the juices. Bring to the boil and cook for 1 minute, stirring. Discard the bay leaf.

10 Pour the sauce into a gravy boat and serve with the gammon, potato cake and broccoli.

American Pork 'n' Beans

*225 g/8 oz/1⅓ cups dried haricot (navy) beans,
soaked overnight in cold water*

450 ml/¾ pt/2 cups water

1 lactose-free pork stock cube

*350 g/12 oz lean belly pork rashers, rinded and diced,
discarding any bones*

1 large onion, finely chopped

1 carrot, finely diced

15 ml/1 tbsp sunflower oil

4 tomatoes, skinned, seeded and chopped

15 ml/1 tbsp black treacle (molasses)

2.5 ml/½ tsp dried mixed herbs

A few drops of Tabasco sauce

5 ml/1 tsp light brown sugar

Salt and freshly ground black pepper

15 ml/1 tbsp chopped fresh parsley, to garnish

Crusty bread (see page 159) and a green salad, to serve

1 Drain the beans and place in a flameproof casserole (Dutch oven) with the measured water. Bring to the boil and boil rapidly for 10 minutes. Stir in the stock cube until dissolved.

2 Meanwhile, brown the pork, onion and carrot in the oil in a frying pan (skillet).

3 Tip into the casserole and add all the remaining ingredients. Stir well.

4 Cover and cook in a preheated oven at 150°C/300°F/ gas mark 2 for 4 hours or until the beans are soft and bathed in a rich sauce. Taste and re-season, if necessary.

5 Sprinkle with parsley and serve with crusty bread and a green salad.

Pork and Prawn Spring Rolls with Egg Fried Rice

SERVES 4

100 g/4 oz pork fillet, cut into very thin strips

15 ml/1 tbsp cornflour (cornstarch)

45 ml/3 tbsp sunflower oil

1 garlic clove, crushed

6 spring onions (scallions), finely chopped

4 mushrooms, thinly sliced

100 g/4 oz beansprouts

50 g/2 oz cooked peeled prawns (shrimp)

1.5 ml/¼ tsp ground ginger

50 g/2 oz frozen peas, thawed

45 ml/3 tbsp soy sauce

4 sheets of filo pastry (paste)

225 g/8 oz/2 cups cooked rice

1 egg, beaten

1 Mix the pork with the cornflour.

2 Heat 15 ml/1 tbsp of the oil in a frying pan (skillet) and fry (sauté) the pork for 1 minute, stirring. Add all the remaining ingredients except for half the peas, 15 ml/1 tbsp of the soy sauce and the pastry, rice and egg and toss for 3 minutes. Leave to cool.

3 Lay the pastry sheets on a work surface and fold into halves. Divide the pork mixture into four and spoon a portion on to the centre of one edge of each sheet.

4 Fold in the sides, then roll up.

5 Brush a baking (cookie) sheet with a little of the remaining oil and place the rolls on the sheet. Brush with a little more of the oil. Bake in a preheated oven at 190°C/375°F/gas mark 5 for about 20 minutes until golden brown.

6 Meanwhile, heat the remaining oil in a frying pan, add the rice and remaining peas and toss until glistening with the oil.

7 Push to one side of the pan and pour the beaten egg into the space. Cook until beginning to set, then gradually draw in the rice until it is marbled with strands of egg. Sprinkle with the remaining soy sauce, toss and serve with the spring rolls.

Curry Turnovers

SERVES 4

1 quantity of Flaky Pastry (see page 169)

1 small onion, finely chopped

1 small eating (dessert) apple, diced

15 g/½ oz/1 tbsp soya spread

25 g/1 oz frozen peas

50 g/2 oz/½ cup cooked roast pork, lamb, chicken or beef, cut into small pieces

5 ml/1 tsp curry powder

15 ml/1 tbsp desiccated (shredded) coconut

5 ml/1 tsp tomato purée (paste)

15 ml/1 tbsp raisins

10 ml/2 tsp water

A little soya milk, to glaze

Mango chutney and salad, to serve

1 Prepare the pastry (paste), then chill while you make the filling.

2 Fry (sauté) the onion and apple in the spread for 2 minutes, stirring, until softened.

3 Stir in all the remaining ingredients and simmer for 5 minutes, stirring occasionally. Remove from the heat and leave to cool.

4 Roll the pastry out to an oblong, fold in three, then roll out and cut into four 18 cm/7 in squares.

5 Spoon the filling into the centres. Brush the edges with water and fold the pastry over to form triangles.

6 Knock up the edges with the back of a knife and make a small hole in the centre of each to allow steam to escape. Transfer to a dampened baking (cookie) sheet and brush with a little soya milk to glaze.

7 Bake in a preheated oven at 200°C/400°F/gas mark 6 for 15–20 minutes until crisp and golden brown.

8 Serve warm or cold with mango chutney and salad.

Chicken Satay with Fresh Pineapple

You can used a drained can of pineapple if fresh is not available.

SERVES 4

1 small onion, finely chopped

1 garlic clove, crushed

15 ml/1 tbsp sunflower oil

30 ml/2 tbsp smooth peanut butter

10 ml/2 tsp lemon juice

15 ml/1 tbsp soy sauce

15 ml/1 tbsp clear honey

1.5 ml/¼ tsp chilli powder

120 ml/4 fl oz/½ cup soya milk

1 small fresh pineapple

450 g/1 lb chicken breasts, cut into cubes

Plain rice and a salad of beansprouts, shredded red (bell) pepper and chopped onion with French dressing, to serve

1   Fry (sauté) the onion and garlic in the oil for 2 minutes until softened.

2   Add all the remaining ingredients except the soya milk, pineapple and chicken. Cook until bubbling, then stir in 90 ml/6 tbsp of the milk. Reduce the heat and simmer for 2 minutes.

3   Meanwhile, cut off the top and base of the pineapple and cut away all the skin. Cut the flesh into thick slices, then cubes.

4   Thread the chicken and pineapple cubes alternately on to wooden skewers that have been soaked in water.

5 Brush all over with a little of the sauce and place on foil on a grill (broiler) rack. Grill (broil) for about 8 minutes, turning occasionally, until cooked through, brushing once with more sauce halfway through cooking.

6 Meanwhile, reheat the remaining sauce with the remaining milk. Serve the Chicken Satay with the remaining sauce, rice and a beansprout, pepper and onion salad.

Smoky Caesar Salad

Remember to check the mustard label carefully.

SERVES 4

---

4 slices of dairy-free French bread

Soya spread, for 'buttering'

2.5 ml/½ tsp garlic salt

45 ml/3 tbsp olive oil

15 ml/1 tbsp white wine vinegar

2.5 ml/½ tsp Dijon mustard

5 ml/1 tsp caster (superfine) sugar

5 ml/1 tsp dried oregano

30 ml/2 tbsp soya yoghurt

1 egg

½ cos (romaine) lettuce, torn into pieces

100 g/4 oz/1 cup smoked tofu, diced

100 g/4 oz/1 small can of smoked oysters or mussels, drained

---

1 Butter the slices of bread with the soya spread and dice. Fry (sauté) the bread cubes in a frying pan (skillet), tossing until golden. Tip into a bowl and sprinkle with the garlic salt.

2 Whisk together the oil, vinegar, mustard, sugar, oregano and garlic, then whisk in the yoghurt.

3 Put the egg in a saucepan, cover with water, bring to the boil and cook for 2 minutes. Rinse under cold water, then carefully remove the shell and mash the egg thoroughly.

4 Put the lettuce in a large bowl. Add the tofu and oysters or mussels and the egg. Pour over the yoghurt dressing and toss thoroughly.

5 Divide between four bowls, sprinkle with the croûtons and serve.

Stuffed Pot Roast Chicken

SERVES 4–6

1.5 kg/3 lb oven-ready chicken

30 ml/2 tbsp fresh dairy-free wholemeal breadcrumbs

100 g/4 oz chicken livers, chopped

1 garlic clove, crushed

45 ml/3 tbsp chopped fresh parsley

Salt and freshly ground black pepper

40 g/1½ oz/3 tbsp soya spread

100 g/4 oz streaky bacon rashers (slices), rinded and diced

2 carrots, diced

2 leeks, sliced

450 g/1 lb whole baby roasting potatoes, scrubbed

15 ml/1 tbsp cornflour (cornstarch)

300 ml/½ pt/1¼ cups lactose-free chicken stock

1 Wipe the chicken inside and out with kitchen paper (paper towels) and pull off any fat just inside the body cavity.

2 Mash the breadcrumbs with the chicken livers, garlic, 30 ml/2 tbsp of the parsley, salt and pepper. Use to stuff the neck end of the bird and secure with cocktail sticks (toothpicks).

3 Melt the spread in a flameproof casserole (Dutch oven) and brown the chicken all over. Remove from the pan.

4 Add the bacon, carrots, leeks and potatoes and toss in the fat. Return the chicken to the pot. Season. Cover and cook in a preheated oven at 180°C/350°F/gas mark 4 for 1½ hours.

5 Transfer the chicken to a carving dish. Lift out the vegetables and keep warm.

6 Blend the cornflour into the cooking juices, then gradually blend in the stock. Bring to the boil and cook for 1 minute, stirring. Taste and re-season, if necessary.

7 Carve the chicken and serve with the vegetables and sauce.

Oven-fried Chicken and Potatoes with Sour Chive Dip

4 chicken portions

45 ml/3 tbsp plain (all-purpose) flour

5 ml/1 tsp curry powder

Salt and freshly ground black pepper

75 g/3 oz/⅓ cup soya spread

75 ml/5 tbsp sunflower oil

450 g/1 lb potatoes, halved and cut into wedges

1.5 ml/¼ tsp chilli powder

150 ml/¼ pt/⅔ cup soya yoghurt

30 ml/2 tbsp snipped fresh chives

A pinch of garlic salt

A mixed salad, to serve

1 Wipe the chicken with kitchen paper (paper towels).

2 Mix the flour with the curry powder and a little salt and pepper. Use to coat the chicken.

3 Melt 50 g/2 oz/¼ cup of the soya spread with 60 ml/ 4 tbsp of the oil in a large roasting tin (pan).

4 Add the chicken portions, skin-sides down.

5 Melt the remaining spread and oil in a separate shallow baking tin. Add the potato wedges, season with salt, pepper and the chilli powder and turn in the fat.

6 Bake the potatoes and chicken in a preheated oven at 180°C/350°F/gas mark 4 for 25 minutes, with the potatoes on the top shelf and the chicken just above the middle.

7 Turn the potatoes and chicken over and return to the oven for a further 25–30 minutes until golden brown and cooked through.

8 Meanwhile, mix the soya yoghurt with the chives, garlic salt and a little pepper. Chill until ready to serve.

9 Drain the chicken and potatoes on kitchen paper and serve with the dip and a mixed salad.

South Pacific Chicken

SERVES 4

4 chicken portions

2.5 ml/½ tsp garlic salt

Freshly ground black pepper

30 ml/2 tbsp sunflower oil

300 ml/½ pt/1¼ cups pineapple juice

2 celery sticks, finely chopped

4 tomatoes, quartered

1 red (bell) pepper, sliced

1 green pepper, sliced

1 green banana, cut into chunks

15 ml/1 tbsp soy sauce

15 ml/1 tbsp cornflour (cornstarch)

30 ml/2 tbsp toasted desiccated (shredded) coconut, to garnish

Plain rice, to serve

1 Wipe the chicken, season with the garlic salt and some pepper and brown in the oil in a flameproof casserole (Dutch oven) on all sides. Cover the pan, reduce the heat and cook gently for 20 minutes.

2 Add the pineapple juice, celery, tomatoes, peppers and banana. Cover again and simmer gently for 20–25 minutes until the chicken is tender.

3 Blend the soy sauce and cornflour together and stir into the liquid, then bring to the boil and cook for 1 minute. Taste and re-season, if necessary.

4 Spoon on to warm plates, sprinkle with toasted coconut and serve with plain rice.

DESSERTS

Desserts can be tricky. You can, of course, enjoy any concoction of fresh fruit you can think of, but many of your more tempting favourites may have dairy produce in them. However, there are quite a lot that don't and in this chapter I've created some wonderful dairy-free alternatives to popular desserts, from a gorgeous lemon cheesecake to a fabulous tiramisu without Mascarpone cheese, and many, many more.

Vanilla Ice

30 ml/2 tbsp cornflour (cornstarch)

100 g/4 oz/½ cup caster (superfine) sugar

300 ml/½ pt/1¼ cups soya milk

1 egg, separated

5 ml/1 tsp vanilla essence (extract)

250 ml/8 fl oz/1 cup Soya Dream (see page 12), chilled

1 Blend the cornflour with the sugar and 30 ml/2 tbsp of the milk in a bowl.

2 Bring the remaining milk to the boil, then whisk into the cornflour mixture. Return to the pan, bring to the boil and cook for 2 minutes, stirring all the time, until thick and smooth. Whisk in the egg yolk and the vanilla essence.

3 Remove from the heat, cover with a circle of wet greaseproof (waxed) paper and leave to cool.

4 Whisk the Soya Dream until thick and doubled in volume. Fold into the custard and turn into a freezer-proof container. Cover and freeze for 2 hours until frozen around the edges.

5 Turn into a bowl and whisk with a fork until smooth.

6 Whisk the egg white until stiff and fold into the mixture with a metal spoon. Return to the container and freeze until firm.

7 Remove from the freezer 10 minutes before serving to soften slightly.

Flavoured Ice Creams

CHOCOLATE ICE

Make as for Vanilla Ice (see page 120), but blend 20 ml/
4 tsp cocoa (unsweetened chocolate) powder with 30 ml/
2 tbsp boiling water and whisk into the hot milk before
blending into the cornflour mixture.

COFFEE ICE

Make as for Vanilla Ice (see page 120), adding 15 ml/1 tbsp
coffee granules to the milk when heating it.

FRUIT ICE

Make as for Vanilla Ice (see page 120). Add 150 ml/¼ pt/
⅔ cup any fruit purée to the partially frozen ice cream
when whisking until smooth, before folding in the egg
white.

FRUIT RIPPLE

Make as for Vanilla Ice (see page 120). Whisk the partially
frozen ice cream until smooth, fold in the egg white, then
fold in 150 ml/¼ pt/⅔ cup fruit purée (raspberry is
particularly good) just until rippled. Turn into the freezer
container and freeze until firm.

Bread and Jam Pudding

For traditional Bread and Butter Pudding, omit the jam (conserve) and layer the buttered bread with 60 ml/4 tbsp sultanas (golden raisins). Dust the top with grated nutmeg instead of flavouring the milk with almond essence (extract).

SERVES 4

4–6 thin slices of dairy-free white bread

50 g/2 oz/¼ cup soya spread

45 ml/3 tbsp raspberry jam

50 g/2 oz/¼ cup granulated sugar

600 ml/1 pt/2½ cups soya milk

2 eggs

A few drops of almond essence (optional)

---

1   Spread the bread with the soya spread and jam.

2   Cut each slice into four triangles.

3   Line a 1.2 litre/2 pt/5 cup ovenproof dish with half the bread. Sprinkle with half the sugar.

4   Arrange the remaining bread triangles attractively on top.

5   Beat the soya milk and eggs together with a few drops of almond essence, if using. Pour over the bread and sprinkle with the remaining sugar.

6   Bake in a preheated oven at 180°C/350°F/gas mark 4 for about 1 hour until golden and set.

Lemon Cheesecake

SERVES 6

50 g/2 oz/¼ cup caster (superfine) sugar

50 g/2 oz/¼ cup soya spread

4 Weetabix

1 lemon jelly (jello) tablet

Boiling water

Finely grated rind and juice of ½ lemon

175 g/6 oz/¾ cup Soft Soya Cheese (see page 183)

1 egg white

Angelica 'leaves' and crystallised (candied) lemon slices, to decorate

1 Put the sugar and soya spread in a saucepan and heat until the fat melts.

2 Crumble in the Weetabix and mix well.

3 Press into the base and sides of a 20 cm/8 in fluted flan dish (pie pan).

4 Bake in a preheated oven at 200°C/400°F/gas mark 6 for 10 minutes. Remove from the oven and leave to cool.

5 Meanwhile, break up the jelly tablet and place in a measuring jug. Make up to 300 ml/½ pt/1¼ cups with boiling water. Stir until the jelly dissolves.

6 Stir in the lemon rind and juice and leave to cool slightly.

7 Whisk in the Soft Soya Cheese. Chill until on the point of setting.

8 Whisk the egg white until stiff and fold in with a metal spoon. Turn into the flan case (pie shell) and chill until set. Decorate with angelica 'leaves' and crystallised lemon slices before serving.

Doughnut Bites

This is a great way of using a loaf that has been reduced in price because it is near its sell-by date (but make sure it is dairy-free, of course!).

SERVES 4–6

---

1 small white uncut loaf of bread

300 ml/½ pt/1¼ cups apple juice

2 eggs, beaten

Oil, for deep-frying

60 ml/4 tbsp caster (superfine) sugar

2.5 ml/½ tsp ground cinnamon

Jam Sauce (see page 181), to serve

1   Cut the crusts off the loaf, then cut the bread into large cubes.

2   Dip first in apple juice, then in beaten egg to coat completely.

3   Heat the oil until a piece of the crust from the loaf browns in 30 seconds. Deep-fry the bread cubes until crisp and golden brown, turning occasionally, if necessary. Drain on kitchen paper (paper towels).

4   Mix the sugar and cinnamon together and toss the cubes in the mixture. Pile the cubes on to plates and trickle the Jam Sauce over. Serve straight away.

Apricot Fool

Ring the changes with other canned fruits.

SERVES 4

---

410 g/14½ oz/1 large can of apricot halves, drained

150 ml/¼ pt/⅔ cup Soya Dream (see page 12), chilled

15 ml/1 tbsp caster (superfine) sugar

Finely grated rind of ½ orange

Toasted flaked (slivered) almonds, to decorate

1 Purée the apricots in a blender or food processor.

2 Whisk the Soya Dream with the sugar until doubled in bulk.

3 Fold the Soya Dream into the apricot purée with the orange rind.

4 Turn into four glass dishes and serve decorated with a few toasted almond flakes.

Peach Filo Tarts

SERVES 4

6 large sheets of filo pastry (paste)

25 g/1 oz/2 tbsp soya spread, melted

Sunflower oil, for greasing

4 peaches, halved, stoned (pitted) and thinly sliced

30 ml/2 tbsp demerara sugar

2.5 ml/½ tsp ground cinnamon

1 Put one sheet of pastry on a work surface and brush with a little of the spread. Place another sheet of pastry on top. Continue to brush and layer all the pastry sheets.

2 Using a saucer as a guide, cut out four rounds from the stack of filo.

3 Transfer to a lightly greased baking (cookie) sheet and brush with any remaining spread.

4 Arrange the peach slices in a starburst pattern on the pastry rounds. Sprinkle with the sugar and cinnamon.

5 Bake in a preheated oven at 200°C/400°F/gas mark 6 for about 20 minutes until golden. Serve warm.

Crème Brûlée

SERVES 4

4 egg yolks

5 ml/1 tsp cornflour (cornstarch)

500 ml/17 fl oz/2¼ cups Soya Dream (see page 12)

2.5 ml/½ tsp vanilla essence (extract)

30 ml/2 tbsp icing (confectioners') sugar

Caster (superfine) sugar

1 Whisk the egg yolks, cornflour and Soya Dream together with the vanilla essence and icing sugar.

2 Place the bowl over a pan of hot water and continue whisking until the mixture coats the back of a spoon.

3 Pour into four individual flameproof dishes and leave to cool, then chill until set.

4 Cover with a thick layer of caster sugar and place under a hot grill (broiler) until the sugar melts and caramelises. Chill again before serving.

Hazelnut Pavlova with Raspberries

SERVES 6

4 egg whites

225 g/8 oz/1 cup caster (superfine) sugar

50 g/2 oz/½ cup ground hazelnuts (filberts)

5 ml/1 tsp vanilla essence (extract)

1.5 ml/¼ tsp cream of tartar

15 ml/1 tbsp white wine vinegar

150 ml/¼ pt/⅔ cup Soya 'Whipped Cream' (see page 186)

350 g/12 oz raspberries

A little icing (confectioners') sugar, for dusting

Toasted chopped hazelnuts, to decorate

1 Whisk the egg whites until stiff. Gradually whisk in the sugar until the mixture forms glistening peaks.

2 Whisk in the ground hazelnuts, vanilla extract, cream of tartar and vinegar.

3 Place a sheet of non-stick baking parchment on a baking (cookie) sheet. Spoon the mixture into a round about 20 cm/8 in in diameter. Make a slight well in the centre.

4 Bake in a preheated oven at 140°C/275°F/gas mark 1 for about 1–1½ hours until a pale biscuit colour on the outside. Remove from the oven and leave to cool.

5 Carefully transfer to a serving plate.

6 Fill the centre with the Soya 'Whipped Cream' and top with the raspberries. Dust with icing sugar, sprinkle with a few toasted, chopped hazelnuts and serve.

Toffee Orange Greengage Pudding

1 orange

50 g/2 oz/¼ cup soya spread

225 g/8 oz/1 cup demerara sugar

15 ml/1 tbsp lemon juice

4 thick slices of dairy-free bread, cut into cubes

450 g/1 lb greengages, halved and stoned (pitted)

Soya yoghurt, to serve

1 Finely grate the rind of the orange, then cut off all the skin and pith and segment the fruit, discarding the membranes.

2 Heat the spread and sugar in a large frying pan (skillet), stirring until melted.

3 Add the lemon juice and orange rind. Stir until completely blended.

4 Add the bread cubes and gently fold into the toffee mixture.

5 Add the greengages and orange segments. Cover and cook gently for about 5 minutes or until the greengages are soft.

6 Spoon into individual bowls and top each with a spoonful of soya yoghurt.

Greek-style Yoghurt with Figs

This is also delicious made with drained, canned figs instead of fresh ones.

SERVES 4

150 ml/¼ pt/⅔ cup Soya Dream (see page 12), chilled

300 ml/½ pt/1¼ cups soya yoghurt

5 ml/1 tsp icing (confectioners') sugar

A few drops of vanilla essence (extract)

4 fresh figs, trimmed and cut into bite-sized pieces

30 ml/2 tbsp brandy (preferably Greek or Spanish) or orange juice

60 ml/4 tbsp clear honey

1 Whisk the Soya Dream until thick and doubled in volume.

2 Gradually whisk in the yoghurt, icing sugar and vanilla essence to taste.

3 Put the figs in the bases of four glass dishes and spoon the brandy or orange juice over.

4 Spoon the yoghurt mixture on top, then spoon the honey over. Chill, if time allows, before serving.

Pear Brûlée

*425 g/15 oz/1 large can of pear quarters, drained,
reserving the juice*

10 ml/2 tsp arrowroot

5 ml/1 tsp lemon juice

150 ml/¼ pt/⅔ cup soya yoghurt

1 large egg

2.5 ml/½ tsp ground cinnamon

45 ml/3 tbsp light brown sugar

1 Put the pear quarters in a 900 ml/1½ pt/3¾ cup ovenproof dish.

2 Blend the arrowroot with a little of the reserved juice in a saucepan, then stir in the remaining pear juice and the lemon juice. Bring to the boil, stirring until thickened and clear. Pour over the pears.

3 Whisk the yoghurt with the egg and cinnamon. Pour over the pears.

4 Bake in a preheated oven at 180°C/350°F/gas mark 4 for about 20 minutes until the custard is set.

5 Sprinkle the top liberally with the sugar and place under a preheated grill (broiler) until the sugar melts and bubbles. Serve hot.

Almost Tiramisu

You don't need the caramel mix included in the packet for this dessert, so try using it for Banana Splits: place a halved banana lengthways in each of four dishes. Put two scoops of Vanilla Ice (see page 120) in the centre. Drizzle with the caramel sauce and serve.

SERVES 6

---

10 dairy-free sponge (lady) fingers

150 ml/¼ pt/⅔ cup strong black coffee

1 packet of crème caramel mix

450 ml/¾ pt/2 cups soya milk

15–30 ml brandy or whisky

1 quantity of Soya 'Whipped Cream' (see page 186)

10 ml/2 tsp cocoa (unsweetened chocolate) powder

15 ml/1 tbsp icing (confectioners') sugar

---

1 Line a 20–23 cm/8–9 in round, shallow serving dish with the sponge fingers. Pour over the coffee and leave to soak.

2 Make up the crème caramel mix with the milk, according to the packet directions. Leave to cool slightly, then stir in the brandy or whisky.

3 Gently pour over the sponge, leave until cold, then chill until set.

4 Meanwhile, make up the Soya 'Whipped Cream' and leave to set. Spread over the top of the pudding. Mix the cocoa and icing sugar together and sift over the surface before serving.

Banana Condé

50 g/2 oz/¼ cup short-grain (pudding) rice

30 ml/2 tbsp cornflour (cornstarch)

600 ml/1 pt/2½ cups soya milk

30 ml/2 tbsp caster (superfine) sugar

4 small ripe bananas

30 ml/2 tbsp apricot jam (conserve)

10 ml/2 tsp lemon juice

2 glacé (candied) cherries, halved

1 Put the rice in a pan and cover with water. Bring to the boil, stirring, reduce the heat and simmer for 15–20 minutes until tender. Drain.

2 Blend the cornflour with a little of the soya milk in a saucepan with the sugar.

3 Blend in the remaining milk and add the rice. Bring to the boil and cook for 2 minutes, stirring all the time, until thickened and smooth. Cover with a circle of wet greaseproof (waxed) paper, to prevent a skin forming, and leave to cool.

4 When cold, spoon half into four sundae glasses. Slice the bananas and put half on top of the rice. Top with the remaining rice and bananas.

5 Heat the jam and lemon juice together and brush over the surface of the bananas.

6 Top each with half a glacé cherry and serve.

Cherries with Kirsch Zabaglione

Instead of the cherries and arrowroot you can, if you prefer, use a can of cherry pie filling, but check that it is lactose-free.

SERVES 4

400 g/14 oz/1 large can of stoned (pitted) black cherries, drained, reserving the juice

10 ml/2 tsp arrowroot

2 eggs

25 g/1 oz/2 tbsp caster (superfine) sugar

45 ml/3 tbsp kirsch

1 Blend a little of the juice from the cherries in a saucepan with the arrowroot. Stir in the remaining juice. Bring to the boil, stirring until thickened and clear. Stir in the cherries.

2 Spoon into four sundae glasses.

3 Put the remaining ingredients in a bowl over a pan of gently simmering water. Whisk with an electric beater or balloon whisk until thick, creamy and voluminous.

4 Spoon over the cherries and serve.

Profiteroles with Dark Chocolate Sauce

1 quantity of Choux Pastry (see page 170)

1 quantity of Soya 'Whipped Cream' (see page 186)

1 quantity of Hot Dark Chocolate Spread
(see page 144), warmed

1 Make up the pastry (paste). Spoon into small balls on a greased baking (cookie) sheet.

2 Bake in a preheated oven at 200°C/400°F/gas mark 6 for about 20 minutes until crisp and golden brown.

3 Transfer to a wire rack, make a slit in the side of each ball to allow steam to escape and leave to cool.

4 Make the Soya 'Whipped Cream'. Spoon into the choux balls and pile into individual dishes.

5 Make the Dark Chocolate Spread and pour over while still warm. Serve straight away.

CHILDREN'S SPECIALS

Children, perhaps more often than
adults, find the restrictions hard to
bear when a food allergy is diagnosed
because they can't have all the
convenience foods that their friends
enjoy. So here are some fantastic
versions of everyday favourites that
I hope will make all the other kids
envious!

Cheese and Tomato Pizza

Vary the toppings for a change: try sweetcorn (corn), sliced or chopped (bell) peppers, sliced mushrooms, anchovies, prawns, tuna, spinach, – whatever your child's (or your!) favourites are. Add them over the tomatoes, and then smear the cheese on top. You can also use chive or garlic and herb flavoured Soya Soft Cheese (see page 183), instead of plain.

SERVES 2–4

1 quantity of Basic Bread Dough (see page 158)

400 g/14 oz/1 large can of chopped tomatoes, well drained

30 ml/2 tbsp tomato purée (paste)

100 g/4 oz/½ cup Soya Soft Cheese

2.5 ml/½ tsp dried oregano

A few black olives

Salt and freshly ground black pepper

6 fresh basil leaves, torn

5 ml/1 tsp olive oil, plus a little for greasing

1 Make up the bread dough. When knocked back (punched down), roll out to a 25 cm/10 in round. Place on an oiled baking (cookie) sheet.

2 Mix the chopped tomatoes and tomato purée together and spread over the surface almost to the edges.

3 Spread the cheese over, then sprinkle with the oregano, scatter the olives on top and season with salt and pepper.

4 Scatter the basil leaves over the surface and drizzle with oil.

5 Bake in a preheated oven at 220°C/425°F/gas mark 7 for 20 minutes until the crust is crisp and golden brown. Serve warm.

Sizzling Peanut Pizza

SERVES 4

Prepare as for Cheese and Tomato Pizza (see page 138), using any toppings you like, but omit the Soya Soft Cheese. Bake for 10 minutes, then spread with a triple quantity of Peanut Rarebit mixture (see page 57) and sprinkle with onion or garlic salt. Cook for a further 10 minutes until the crust is crisp and serve warm.

Crispy Beef Pancakes

SERVES 4

1 quantity of Simple Pancakes (see page 173)

425 g/15 oz/1 large can of minced (ground) steak in gravy

2 eggs, beaten

75 g/3 oz/1½ cups fresh dairy-free white breadcrumbs

Oil, for shallow-frying

1 Make up the pancakes.

2 Divide the steak in gravy between the pancakes. Brush all round the edges with beaten egg.

3 Fold in the sides of the pancakes, then the ends, over the filling to form parcels.

4 Brush each with beaten egg, then coat in breadcrumbs. Repeat the brushing and coating. Chill for 30 minutes.

5 Shallow-fry in hot oil for about 3 minutes on each side until golden brown and piping hot. Drain on kitchen paper (paper towels).

Chicken Dippers

Use turkey steaks instead of chicken for a change.

SERVES 4

30 ml/2 tbsp plain (all-purpose) flour

Salt and freshly ground black pepper

5 ml/1 tsp dried onion granules

100 g/4 oz/1 cup self-raising (self-rising) flour

About 150 ml/¼ pt/⅔ cup water

4 skinless chicken breasts, cut into bite-sized pieces

30 ml/2 tbsp soya milk

Oil, for shallow-frying

Barbecue Sauce (see page 181), to serve

1 Mix the plain flour on a plate with a little salt and pepper and the onion granules.

2 Sift the self-raising flour into a bowl. Add a good pinch of salt. Mix with the cold water to form a thick cream.

3 Dip the pieces of chicken in the milk, then in the plain flour mixture.

4 Heat about 5 mm/¼ in oil in a large frying pan (skillet). Dip the chicken pieces in the batter and shallow-fry, turning once, for about 6 minutes until crisp, golden and cooked through. Drain on kitchen paper (paper towels) and serve with Barbecue Sauce for dipping.

Mini Kievs

50 g/2 oz/¼ cup soya spread

1 small garlic clove, crushed

2.5 ml/½ tsp dried mixed herbs

Salt and freshly ground black pepper

350 g/12 oz turkey steaks or boneless chicken thighs, minced (ground)

2 eggs, beaten

30 ml/2 tbsp plain (all-purpose) flour

50 g/2 oz/1 cup fresh dairy-free white breadcrumbs

Oil, for shallow-frying

1 Mash the soya spread with the garlic, herbs and a little salt and pepper. Shape into a roll on a piece of greaseproof (waxed) paper and roll up in the paper. Freeze until firm.

2 Mix the minced turkey or chicken with one of the eggs and a little salt and pepper. Divide into 12 pieces.

3 Put the remaining egg in one shallow dish and the breadcrumbs in another.

4 Cut the frozen garlic 'butter' into 12 pieces. Flatten each portion of mince and put a piece of the 'butter' in the centre. Wrap up completely and roll in the flour. Coat in beaten egg, then breadcrumbs to cover thoroughly. Chill, if time allows, before cooking.

5 Heat about 5 mm/¼ in oil in a large frying pan (skillet). Shallow-fry the balls for about 6 minutes, turning once or twice, until golden brown and cooked through. Drain on kitchen paper (paper towels) and serve straight away.

Funky Fish Cakes

If you don't have time to poach fresh tomatoes, use a
410 g/15 oz/large can of plum tomatoes instead.

SERVES 4

225 g/8 oz potatoes, cut into chunks

225 g/8 oz white fish fillet, skinned and any bones removed

100 g/4 oz bacon pieces, rinded

25 g/1 oz/2 tbsp soya spread

15 ml/1 tbsp snipped fresh chives

Salt and freshly ground black pepper

3 eggs

75 g/3 oz/¾ cup dried dairy-free breadcrumbs

Flour, for dusting

Oil, for shallow-frying

8 tomatoes

60 ml/4 tbsp water

A sprig of fresh mint

Peas, to serve

1 Put the potatoes in a saucepan of lightly salted water and bring to the boil.

2 Place the fish in a steamer or colander over the pan of potatoes. Cover and cook for about 10 minutes until the fish and potatoes are tender. Remove the fish. Drain the potatoes and place in a bowl. Add the fish and mash the potatoes and fish together.

3 Meanwhile, fry (sauté) the bacon in the soya spread for 2 minutes. Snip the bacon into small pieces with scissors, then add to the potato mixture, together with the melted spread in the pan.

4 Add the chives and a little salt and pepper and mix well. Beat one of the eggs and add to the mixture to bind.

5 Beat the remaining eggs in a shallow dish. Put the breadcrumbs in a separate dish.

6 Dust your hands with flour, then shape the mixture into eight fish-shaped cakes.

7 Dip the cakes in the beaten egg, then the breadcrumbs, until thoroughly coated. Chill for at least 30 minutes, if possible.

8 Make a cross-cut in the top of each tomato. Place in a saucepan with the water and mint. Bring to the boil, reduce the heat, cover and cook very gently for about 5 minutes until the tomatoes are soft but still hold their shape.

9 Shallow-fry the cakes in hot oil for about 2 minutes on each side, until golden brown. Drain on kitchen paper (paper towels).

10 Transfer the fish cakes to warm plates. Serve with the poached tomatoes and peas.

Dark Chocolate Balls

When warmed, the mixture makes a delicious Dark Chocolate Spread for sandwiches and cakes.

MAKES 16
---

15 g/½ oz/1 tbsp soya spread

15 g/½ oz/1 tbsp hard white vegetable fat

15 ml/1 tbsp cornflour (cornstarch)

30 ml/2 tbsp cocoa (unsweetened chocolate) powder

30 ml/2 tbsp caster (superfine) sugar

15 ml/1 tbsp hot water

Oil, for greasing

Extra cocoa powder or coloured sprinkles, to decorate

1 Put the fats, cornflour, cocoa and sugar in a saucepan and heat gently, stirring, for about 2 minutes until melted and blended.

2 Beat in the water and cook for 1 minute.

3 Oil a small metal plate and spoon the chocolate mixture on to it. Spread out to a fairly thin layer.

4 Leave to cool, then chill. When fairly firm, divide into 16 pieces and roll into small balls. Roll in cocoa powder or coloured sprinkles and store in the fridge.

Knickerbocker Glory

1 strawberry or raspberry jelly (jello) tablet

8 dairy-free sponge (lady) fingers

30 ml/2 tbsp pure orange juice

225 g/8 oz raspberries or strawberries, sliced

4 scoops of Vanilla Ice (see page 120)

150 ml/¼ pt/⅔ cup sweetened Soya 'Whipped Cream' (see page 186)

Toasted chopped nuts and coloured sprinkles, to decorate

1 Make up the jelly according to packet directions and leave to set. Chop up.

2 Break up the sponge fingers and place in a bowl. Sprinkle with the orange juice and leave to soak.

3 Spoon the soaked sponges into four tall sundae glasses. Top with half the chopped jelly.

4 Cover with the fruit, then the Vanilla Ice and finally the remaining chopped jelly.

5 Top with Soya 'Whipped Cream' and decorate with nuts and coloured sprinkles.

Chocolate Cream Buns

1 quantity of Choux Pastry (see page 170)

1 quantity of Soya 'Whipped Cream' (see page 186)

90 ml/6 tbsp icing (confectioners') sugar

15 ml/1 tbsp cocoa (unsweetened chocolate) powder

Cold water, to mix

1 Make up the pastry (paste) and place in four round piles on a greased baking (cookie) sheet.

2 Bake in a preheated oven at 200°C/400°F/gas mark 6 for about 30 minutes until risen and golden brown.

3 Transfer to a wire rack to cool. When cool, gently split the sides and scoop out any uncooked dough.

4 Fill with the Soya 'Whipped Cream'. Place on individual plates.

5 Mix the icing sugar with the cocoa powder and then blend in cold water, a small spoonful at a time, until the mixture has the consistency of thick cream. Spread over the buns and serve cold.

Jam Doughnuts

1 quantity of Milk Bread dough (see page 160)

50 ml/10 tsp any red jam (conserve)

Sunflower oil, for greasing and deep-frying

100 g/4 oz/½ cup caster (superfine) sugar, for dusting

1 Make the dough and leave to rise as directed in the recipe.

2 Knock back (punch down) the dough and divide into 10 pieces.

3 Flatten each to a round and put 5 ml/1 tsp jam in the centre of each. Draw the dough up round the jam to form a ball, pressing the edges firmly together to seal.

4 Put on a greased baking (cookie) sheet and leave to rise for about 15 minutes until doubled in size.

5 Heat the oil until a cube of day-old bread browns in 30 seconds. Cook the doughnuts for about 6 minutes until golden brown and cooked through, gently turning in the oil, if necessary.

6 Drain on kitchen paper (paper towels).

7 Put the sugar in a plastic bag, drop in one doughnut at a time and shake the bag to coat the doughnut in sugar. Repeat with the remaining doughnuts. Serve warm or cold.

Cinnamon Ring Doughnuts

1 quantity of Milk Bread dough (see page 160)

Oil, for greasing and deep-frying

100 g/4 oz/½ cup caster (superfine) sugar

10 ml/2 tsp ground cinnamon

1　Make the dough and leave to rise as directed in the recipe.

2　Knock back (punch down) and divide the dough into 12 pieces.

3　Roll out each piece to a sausage shape and draw the ends round to form a ring. Press the edges well together to seal.

4　Place on a greased baking (cookie) sheet and leave in a warm place for about 15 minutes until doubled in bulk.

5　Heat the oil until a cube of day-old bread browns in 30 seconds and cook the doughnut rings for about 5 minutes until golden and cooked through. Drain on kitchen paper (paper towels).

6　Mix the sugar and cinnamon together in a plastic bag. Add one doughnut one at a time and shake the bag well to coat in the sugar mixture. Repeat with the remaining doughnuts. Serve warm or cold.

Marshmallow Dream Cake

Sunflower oil, for greasing

75 g/3 oz/⅓ cup soya spread

75 g/3 oz/⅓ cup caster (superfine) sugar

A few drops of vanilla essence (extract)

2 eggs, beaten

75 g/3 oz/¾ cup self-raising (self-rising) flour

15 g/½ oz/2 tbsp cornflour (cornstarch)

100 g/4 oz pink and white marshmallows

45 ml/3 tbsp raspberry jam (conserve)

1 Grease and line a 15 cm/6 in deep, round cake tin (pan) with greased greaseproof (waxed) paper.

2 Cream the soya spread and sugar together with a few drops of vanilla essence until light and fluffy. Add the eggs, a little at a time, beating well after each addition.

3 Sift the flour and cornflour over the surface and fold in with a metal spoon.

4 Turn the mixture into the prepared tin and cook in a preheated oven at 190°C/375°F/gas mark 5 for about 45 minutes until risen and golden and a skewer inserted in the centre comes out clean.

5 Meanwhile, snip the marshmallows in half with scissors, dipped in warm water. As soon as the cake is cooked, cover the surface with the marshmallows, cut sides down, and leave to cool in the tin. The marshmallows will melt slightly and stick to the cake.

6 When cold, remove the cake from the tin and discard the paper. Split in half and sandwich back together with raspberry jam.

Digestive Biscuits

100 g/4 oz/1 cup wholemeal self-raising (self-rising) flour

100 g/4 oz/1 cup self-raising flour

A pinch of salt

150 g/5 oz/⅔ cup soya spread

100 g/4 oz/½ cup caster (superfine) sugar

Flour, for dusting

1 Mix the flours in a bowl with the salt.

2 Add the soya spread and sugar and work together with a wooden spoon to form a dough.

3 Knead together into a ball and wrap in a plastic bag. Chill for 30 minutes.

4 Roll out thinly on a lightly floured surface and cut into rounds using a 7.5 cm/3 in biscuit (cookie) cutter.

5 Place on lightly greased baking (cookie) sheets and prick with a fork.

6 Bake in a preheated oven at 180°C/350°F/gas mark 4 for 20 minutes until golden. Leave to cool on the sheets for a few minutes, then transfer to a wire rack to cool completely. Store in an airtight container.

Chocolate Digestives

MAKES ABOUT 24

1 quantity of Digestive Biscuits (see page 150)

3 quantities of Dark Chocolate Spread (see page 144)

1 Prepare and cook the biscuits (cookies) and leave to cool.

2 Make up the Dark Chocolate Spread and, while still warm, spread thinly over the base of the biscuits and decorate with the prongs of a fork. Leave chocolate-side up on the cooling rack to set.

Gingerbread Men

MAKES 12

225 g/8 oz/2 cups plain (all-purpose) flour

1.5 ml/¼ tsp salt

2.5 ml/½ tsp bicarbonate of soda (baking soda)

2.5 ml/½ tsp ground ginger

1.5 ml/¼ tsp ground cinnamon

50 g/2 oz/¼ cup soya spread

100 g/4 oz/½ cup light brown sugar

30 ml/2 tbsp black treacle (molasses)

45 ml/3 tbsp soya milk

A few currants and glacé (candied) cherries

75 g/3 oz/½ cup icing (confectioners') sugar, sifted

10 ml/2 tsp water

1 Sift the flour, salt, bicarbonate of soda and spices into a bowl.

2 Put the soya spread, sugar, treacle and milk in a saucepan and heat gently until the fat melts.

3 Pour into the dry ingredients and mix to form a firm dough. Leave to cool, then chill for 30 minutes.

4 Roll out the dough on a lightly floured surface to about 5 mm/¼ in thick. Cut into 12 shapes, using a gingerbread-man cutter. Place the men well apart on greased baking (cookie) sheets. Press in currants for eyes and buttons and pieces of cherry for mouths.

5 Bake in a preheated oven at 160°C/325°F/gas mark 3 for 20 minutes. Cool slightly, then transfer to a wire rack to cool completely.

6 When cold, mix the icing sugar with the water to a smooth cream. Place in a piping bag fitted with a plain tube (tip), or in a paper piping bag with the point snipped off, and pipe bow ties, collars, cuffs, etc. on the men. Leave to set. Store in an airtight container.

Toffee Apples

I use 5 mm/¼ in thick pieces of dowelling, cut into 15 cm/ 6 in lengths, for the sticks, but you could improvise with wooden chopsticks!

MAKES 8

8 small eating (dessert) apples

450 g/1 lb/2 cups demerara sugar

50 g/2 oz/¼ cup soya spread

10 ml/2 tsp malt vinegar

150 ml/¼ pt/⅔ cup water

15 ml/1 tbsp golden (light corn) syrup

1 Wash the apples and dry on kitchen paper (paper towels). Push a stick into each core to hold the fruit firmly.

2 Put the remaining ingredients in a heavy-based saucepan. Melt very slowly over a gentle heat until the sugar has completely dissolved, stirring occasionally.

3 Bring to the boil and boil to 145°C/290°F (use a sugar thermometer) or until the mixture is golden brown and a small spoonful forms a hard but not brittle ball when dropped into a cup of cold water.

4 Quickly dip the apples in the hot toffee to coat completely, twirl round for a few seconds to distribute the toffee evenly, then transfer to non-stick baking parchment on a baking (cookie) sheet, to set.

Teacup Honey Fluff Nougat

*Ring the changes by adding dried mixed fruit (fruit cake mix)
instead of the nuts, cherries and angelica. You can also add
15 ml/1 tbsp cocoa (unsweetened chocolate) powder to the
sugar to make Chocolate Nougat.*

MAKES ABOUT 25 PIECES

---

1 teacup granulated sugar

½ teacup thick honey

5 ml/1 tsp water

5 ml/1 tsp lemon juice

A good pinch of cream of tartar

2.5 ml/½ tsp vanilla essence (extract)

1 egg white

30 ml/2 tbsp chopped mixed nuts

15 ml/1 tbsp glacé (candied) cherries, chopped

15 ml/1 tbsp chopped angelica

---

1 Put the sugar, honey, water and lemon juice in a heavy-
   based saucepan. Heat gently, stirring, until the sugar
   has dissolved.

2 Stir in the cream of tartar and vanilla essence and boil
   for about 2 minutes to 115°C/242°F (use a sugar
   thermometer) or until the mixture forms a soft ball
   when a teaspoonful is dropped into a cup of cold water.
   Turn down the heat as low as possible to prevent
   setting yet.

3 Whisk the egg whites until stiff.

4 Pour the fudge mixture on to the egg white. Add the
   nuts, cherries and angelica and whisk until the mixture
   is thick and creamy.

5 Pour into an oiled 18 cm/7 in shallow baking tin (pan) and leave to cool. When almost cold, cut into pieces. When completely cold, remove from the tin, wrap each piece in clingfilm (plastic wrap) and store in an airtight container.

Buttery Crispy Popcorn

MAKES 1 LARGE BOWL

40 g/1½ oz/3 tbsp soya spread

50 g/2 oz/½ cup popping corn (maize)

45 ml/3 tbsp golden (light corn) syrup

1 Melt 25 g/1 oz/2 tbsp of the soya spread in a large non-stick saucepan with a lid.

2 Add the corn, cover with the lid, shake the pan vigorously and cook over a moderate heat. The corn will start to pop. Hold the lid on firmly and shake the pan from time to time until all the popping stops.

3 Remove the lid and add the remaining spread and the syrup. Cook over a gentle heat, stirring all the time, for 3–4 minutes until each piece of corn is coated stickily and the mixture is hot but not burning.

4 Tip into a large bowl and leave to cool. Leftovers – if there are any! – can be stored in an airtight container.

Chocolate Smoothie

Make this extra-special by adding a scoop of Vanilla or Chocolate Ice (see pages 120–1).

SERVES 1

7.5 ml/1½ tsp cocoa (unsweetened chocolate) powder

15 ml/1 tbsp boiling water

1 ripe banana

150 ml/¼ pt/⅔ cup cold soya milk

2 ice cubes

---

1 Blend the cocoa powder with the water and put in a blender or food processor with the banana. Run the machine until smooth.

2 Add the milk and ice cubes and run the machine again until thick and frothy.

3 Pour into a glass and serve.

BREADS, BISCUITS, CAKES AND PASTRIES

Milk and other dairy produce have a nasty habit of creeping into commercially made breads, biscuits (cookies) and cakes in all kinds of different disguises. However, this chapter contains a whole selection of great recipes that have not so much been glanced at by a cow!

Basic Bread Dough

*This quantity of dough will also make one large pizza
(see pages 138–9)*

MAKES 1 SMALL LOAF (SEE PAGE 159)

---

225 g/8 oz/2 cups strong plain (bread) flour

2.5 ml/½ tsp salt

10 ml/2 tsp easy-blend dried yeast

15 ml/1 tbsp olive oil

150 ml/¼ pt/⅔ cup hand-hot water

Flour, for dusting

---

1 Mix the flour, salt and yeast in a bowl.

2 Stir in the oil and mix with the water to form a soft but not sticky dough.

3 Knead on a lightly floured surface for several minutes until smooth and elastic.

4 Place in a lightly oiled plastic bag and leave in a warm place for about 45 minutes until doubled in bulk.

5 Knock back (punch down) and use as required.

Crusty Loaf

MAKES 1 LOAF

1 quantity of Basic Bread Dough (see page 158)

Oil, for greasing

Beaten egg or soya milk, to glaze

5 ml/1 tsp poppy, sesame or caraway seeds (optional)

1 Make the dough, leave to rise, then knock back (punch down).

2 Lightly oil a 450 g/1lb loaf tin (pan). Shape the dough into an oblong and place in the tin. Leave in a warm place for about 30 minutes until the dough reaches the top of the tin.

3 Gently brush the top with egg or soya milk and sprinkle with seeds, if liked.

4 Bake in a preheated oven at 220°C/425°F/gas mark 7 for about 20 minutes or until crisp and golden.

5 Tip the bread out of the tin and tap the base – it should sound hollow. Put the loaf directly on the oven shelf and bake for a further 5 minutes to crisp the base. Cool on a wire rack.

Milk Bread

MAKES 1 LOAF

450 g/1 lb/4 cups strong plain (bread) flour

5 ml/1 tsp salt

10 ml/2 tsp easy-blend dried yeast

20 g/¾ oz/1½ tbsp soya spread, melted

300 ml/½ pt/1¼ cups hand-hot soya milk

1 small egg, beaten

Flour, for dusting

A little extra soya milk, to glaze

A little oil, for greasing

1 Sift the flour and salt into a bowl. Stir in the yeast.

2 Make a well in the centre and add the melted soya spread, soya milk and egg. Mix with a wooden spoon to form a dough, then draw together with your hand, kneading until smooth and elastic.

3 Cover with lightly greased clingfilm (plastic wrap) and leave in a warm place for about 45 minutes until doubled in bulk.

4 Knock back (punch down) and knead briefly in a lightly floured surface. Shape into an oval and place in a lightly greased 900 g/2 lb loaf tin (pan) and leave in a warm place until the dough reaches the top of the tin.

5 Brush with a little soya milk to glaze, and bake in a preheated oven at 230°C/450°F/gas mark 8 for about 20–25 minutes until the top is golden brown and the base sounds hollow when the loaf is tipped out and tapped. Cool on a wire rack.

Garlic Bread

1 small dairy-free French stick

75 g/3 oz/⅓ cup soya spread

1 large garlic clove, crushed

15 ml/1 tbsp chopped fresh parsley

Salt and freshly ground black pepper

1 Cut the bread into 12 slices, not quite through the bottom crust.

2 Mash the soya spread with the garlic, parsley and a little salt and pepper and spread between each slice. Smear any remainder over the top.

3 Wrap in foil, sealing the edges well, and bake in a preheated oven at 200°C/400°F/gas mark 6 for about 15 minutes until the crust feels crisp when gently squeezed (wear an oven glove!).

Quick Sun-dried Tomato and Olive Rolls

MAKES 8

375 g/13 oz/3¼ cups strong plain (bread) flour, plus extra for dusting

2.5 ml/½ tsp salt

1 vitamin C tablet, crushed

30 ml/2 tbsp olive oil

10 ml/2 tsp easy-blend dried yeast

5 ml/1 tsp caster (superfine) sugar

5 sun-dried tomatoes, chopped

30 ml/2 tbsp stoned (pitted) black olives, sliced

250 ml/8 fl oz/1 cup hand-hot water

A little soya yoghurt, to glaze

1 Mix the flour with the salt in a large bowl.

2 Stir in all the remaining ingredients except the water.

3 Gradually add enough water to form a soft but not sticky dough.

4 Knead gently on a lightly floured surface for 5 minutes until smooth and elastic.

5 Shape into eight rolls and place well apart on a lightly oiled baking (cookie) sheet. Brush with soya yoghurt to glaze.

6 Bake in a preheated oven at 200°C/400°F/gas mark 6 for 20 minutes until risen and golden and the bases sound hollow when tapped.

Quick Walnut Rolls

MAKES 8

Prepare as for Quick Sun-dried Tomato and Olive Rolls (see page 162), but substitute 50 g/2 oz/½ cup chopped walnuts for the tomatoes and olives and add 15 ml/1 tbsp snipped fresh chives.

Herb and Sunflower Seed Bread

SERVES 4

1 small dairy-free wholemeal French stick

75 g/3 oz/⅓ cup soya spread

15 ml/1 tbsp chopped fresh parsley

15 ml/1 tbsp chopped fresh marjoram

30 ml/2 tbsp sunflower seeds

2.5 ml/½ tsp celery salt

Freshly ground black pepper

1 Cut the bread into 12 slices, not quite through the bottom crust.

2 Mash the soya spread with the herbs, seeds, celery salt and a good grinding of pepper.

3 Spread between the slices and spread any remainder over the top.

4 Wrap in foil, sealing the edges well and bake in a preheated oven at 200°C/400°F/gas mark 6 for about 15 minutes until the crust feels crisp when gently squeezed (it will be very hot, so use an oven-glove).

Plain Yoghurt Scones

To make Sweet Yoghurt Scones, add 15 ml/1 tbsp caster (superfine) sugar to the mixture.

MAKES 6–8

225 g/8 oz/2 cups self-raising (self-rising) flour

A pinch of salt

50 g/2 oz/¼ cup soya spread, plus extra for 'buttering'

75 ml/5 tbsp soya yoghurt

About 45 ml/3 tbsp soya milk, plus extra for glazing

1 Sift the flour and salt into a bowl.

2 Add the measured spread and rub in with your fingertips until the mixture resembles breadcrumbs.

3 Stir in the yoghurt and enough soya milk to form a soft but not sticky dough.

4 Knead gently into a round and pat out to about 2 cm/ ¾ in thick. Cut into six or eight scones (biscuits) using a biscuit (cookie) cutter.

5 Transfer to a non-stick baking (cookie) sheet and brush with a little soya milk.

6 Bake in a preheated oven at 230°C/450°F/gas mark 8 for about 12 minutes until well risen and golden and the bases sound hollow when tapped.

7 Serve warm, split and buttered.

Fruit Scones

MAKES 6–8

Prepare as for Plain or Sweet Yoghurt Scones (above), but add 30 ml/2 tbsp sultanas (golden raisins) to the dry mixture before adding the yoghurt and milk.

Jam and 'Cream' Sponge

SERVES 8

---

225 g/8 oz/1 cup soya spread

175 g/6 oz/¾ cup caster (superfine) sugar

175 g/6 oz/1½ cups self-raising (self-rising) flour

5 ml/1 tsp baking powder

2.5 ml/½ tsp vanilla essence (extract)

3 eggs

100 g/4 oz/⅔ cup icing (confectioners') sugar, plus extra for dusting

45 ml/3 tbsp raspberry jam (conserve)

1 Grease and line the bases of two 18 cm/7 in round sandwich tins (pans) with greased greaseproof (waxed) paper.

2 Put 175 g/6 oz/¾ cup of the soya spread in a food processor with the sugar, flour, baking powder, vanilla essence and eggs and run the machine until just smooth – no longer. Alternatively, place in a bowl and beat with a wooden spoon until smooth.

3 Divide between the tins and smooth the surfaces. Bake in a preheated oven at 190°C/375°F/gas mark 5 for 20 minutes or until risen and golden and the centres spring back when lightly pressed.

4 Cool slightly, then turn out on to a wire rack, remove the paper and leave to cool completely.

5 To make the 'cream', put the remaining spread in a bowl. Sift the icing sugar over. Beat with a wooden spoon until smooth and fluffy.

6 Sandwich the cakes together with the 'cream' and jam. Place on a serving plate and sift a little icing sugar over the surface.

Black Forest Gâteau

SERVES 8

225 g/8 oz/1 cup soya spread

175 g/6 oz/¾ cup caster (superfine) sugar

160 g/5½ oz/scant 1½ cups self-raising (self-rising) flour

20 g/¾ oz/3 tbsp cocoa (unsweetened chocolate) powder

10 ml/2 tsp baking powder

3 eggs

100 g/4 oz/⅔ cup icing (confectioners') sugar, plus extra for dusting

45 ml/3 tbsp black cherry jam (conserve)

1 Grease and line the bases of two 18 cm/7 in sandwich tins (pans) with greased greaseproof (waxed) paper.

2 Put 175 g/6 oz/¾ cup of the soya spread in a food processor with the sugar. Sift the flour, 15 g/½ oz/2 tbsp of the cocoa powder and the baking powder over the surface. Add the eggs and process until the mixture is just smooth. Alternatively, put the ingredients in a bowl and beat with a wooden spoon until smooth.

3 Divide between the tins and smooth the surfaces.

4 Bake in a preheated oven at 190°C/375°F/gas mark 5 for 20 minutes or until risen and the centres spring back when lightly pressed. Cool slightly, then turn out on to a wire rack, remove the paper and leave to cool.

5 Put the remaining spread in a bowl. Sift the icing sugar and remaining cocoa powder over the surface. Beat with a wooden spoon until smooth and fluffy.

6 Sandwich the cakes together with the jam and chocolate 'cream' and dust with a little icing sugar.

Everyday Fruit Cake

SERVES 8

175 g/6 oz/¾ cup soya spread, plus extra for greasing

175 g/6 oz/¾ cup caster (superfine) sugar

3 eggs

225 g/8 oz/2 cups plain (all-purpose) flour

5 ml/1 tsp mixed (apple-pie) spice

225 g/8 oz/2 cups dried mixed fruit (fruit cake mix)

15–30 ml/1–2 tbsp soya milk

1 Grease and line an 18 cm/7 in deep, round cake tin (pan) with greased greaseproof (waxed) paper.

2 Beat the soya spread and sugar together until light and fluffy.

3 Add the eggs one at a time, beating well after each addition. If the mixture curdles, beat in 30 ml/2 tbsp of the flour.

4 Sift the flour and spice over the surface. Fold in with a metal spoon.

5 Fold in the fruit and add milk, as necessary, to give a soft, dropping consistency. It should not be too wet.

6 Turn into the prepared tin and level the surface. Bake in a preheated oven at 160°C/325°F/gas mark 3 for about 1¼ hours until the top is golden brown and a skewer inserted in the centre comes out clean.

7 Cool slightly, then turn out on to a wire rack, remove the paper and leave to cool. Store in an airtight container.

Shortcrust Pastry

MAKES 175 G/6 OZ

65 g/2½ oz/generous ¼ cup soya spread

15 ml/1 tbsp water

100 g/4 oz/1 cup plain (all-purpose) flour

A pinch of salt

1 Put the soya spread in a bowl. Add the water and 25 g/ 1 oz/¼ cup of the flour.

2 Mix with a fork to a smooth paste.

3 Work in the remaining flour and salt to form a soft dough.

4 Wrap and chill the pastry (paste) for 30 minutes before using.

Flaky Pastry

100 g/4 oz/1 cup plain (all-purpose) flour

A pinch of salt

25 g/1 oz/2 tbsp soya spread

30–45 ml/2–3 tbsp iced water

50 g/2 oz/¼ cup hard white vegetable fat

1 Sift the flour and salt into a bowl. Add the soya spread and rub in with your fingertips.

2 Mix with enough iced water to form a soft but not sticky dough.

3 Roll out the dough to an oblong. Cut half the fat into thumbnail-sized pieces and dot over two-thirds of the dough. Fold the 'undotted' third of the dough down over the fat and the other third up over the top. Press the edges together and give the dough a quarter turn.

4 Roll out to an oblong and repeat the process with the remaining fat. Seal, roll and fold once more, then wrap and chill for 30 minutes.

5 When ready to use, roll and fold once more, then roll out to about 5 mm/¼ in thick and use as required.

Choux Pastry

MAKES ENOUGH FOR 1 GOUGÈRE OR PROFITEROLES TO SERVE 4

65 g/2½ oz/scant ¾ cup plain (all-purpose) flour

A pinch of salt

150 ml/¼ pt/⅔ cup water

50 g/2 oz/¼ cup soya spread

2 eggs, beaten

1 Sift the flour and salt on to a sheet of kitchen paper (paper towel).

2 Put the water and soya spread in a saucepan and heat until the fat melts.

3 Add the sifted flour all in one go and beat with a wooden spoon until the mixture leaves the sides of the pan clean.

4 Remove from the heat and gradually add the eggs, a little at a time, beating well after each addition until the mixture is smooth and glossy but still holds its shape. Use immediately as required.

Maids of Honour

Use currants instead of the mixed fruit, if you prefer.

MAKES 10

1 quantity of Flaky Pastry (see page 169)

75 g/3 oz/⅓ cup Soft Soya Cheese (see page 183)

20 g/¾ oz/2 tbsp dried mixed fruit (fruit cake mix)

10 g/2 tsp soya spread

25 g/1 oz/2 tbsp caster (superfine) sugar

Finely grated rind of ½ lemon

15 g/½ oz/2 tbsp ground almonds

1 egg, beaten

A little sifted icing (confectioners') sugar, to decorate

1 Make the pastry (paste) and chill, then roll and fold once more. Roll out and cut into 10 rounds using a 7.5 cm/3 in biscuit (cookie) cutter. Use to line the sections of a tartlet tin (patty pan).

2 Beat all the remaining ingredients together and use to fill the pastry cases (pie shells).

3 Bake in a preheated oven at 190°C/375°F/gas mark 5 for 35 minutes until risen and golden brown.

4 Transfer to a wire rack to cool, then dust with sifted icing sugar before serving.

Yorkshire Pudding

SERVES 4

100 g/4 oz/1 cup plain (all-purpose) flour

Salt and freshly ground black pepper

2 eggs

150 ml/¼ pt/⅔ cup soya milk

150 ml/¼ pt/⅔ cup water

Oil, for greasing

1   Sift the flour and a pinch of salt into a bowl. Add a good grinding of pepper.

2   Make a well in the centre and add the eggs. Pour in half the soya milk and water.

3   Beat with a wooden spoon or balloon whisk until the mixture forms a thick, smooth batter. Stir in the remaining milk and water.

4   Pour in enough oil to coat the bases of each of 12 sections of a tartlet tin (patty pan) or an 18 × 28 cm/7 × 11 in shallow baking tin (pan). Heat towards the top of a preheated oven at 220°C/425°F/gas mark 7 until sizzling.

5   Give the batter a final whisk, pour into the sizzling oil and bake for about 20 minutes for small puddings, 35 minutes for large, until risen, crisp and golden.

Simple Pancakes

You can serve these hot with sugar and lemon, or stuff with a savoury filling or canned or fresh fruit and Vanilla Ice (see page 120).

MAKES 8

---

100 g/4 oz/1 cup plain (all-purpose) flour

A pinch of salt

1 egg

300 ml/½ pt/1¼ cups soya milk

15 g/½ oz/1 tbsp soya spread, melted

Oil, for cooking

1 Sift the flour and salt into a bowl.

2 Make a well in the centre and add the egg and half the soya milk. Beat well to form a thick batter.

3 Stir in the remaining soya milk and the soya spread. Leave to stand for 30 minutes before using, if time allows.

4 Heat a little oil in a frying pan (skillet) and pour off the excess. Add just enough batter to coat the base of the pan when swirled round. Cook until the underside is brown and the top is just set.

5 Toss or flip over with a palette knife and cook the other side quickly. Slide out of the pan and keep warm, either on a plate over a pan of gently simmering water or in the oven, while cooking the remainder. Use as required.

Fork Biscuits

65 g/2½ oz/scant ⅓ cup soya spread

50 g/2 oz/¼ cup caster (superfine) sugar

5 ml/1 tsp vanilla essence (extract)

100 g/4 oz/1 cup self-raising (self-rising) flour

Oil, for greasing

Whole blanched almonds or halved glacé (candied) cherries, to decorate

1　Put all the ingredients in a bowl and work with a fork until the mixture is completely blended and forms a ball.

2　Roll into walnut-sized balls and place a little apart on a lightly greased baking (cookie) sheet (you may need two).

3　Press down each ball with a fork dipped in cold water.

4　Bake in a preheated oven at 190°C/375°F/gas mark 5 for about 15 minutes until pale golden brown. Top each immediately with a nut or half a cherry and transfer to a wire rack to cool. Store in an airtight container.

Chocolate Fork Biscuits

MAKES ABOUT 20

Prepare as for Fork Biscuits (above) but substitute 15 ml/ 1 tbsp of the flour with cocoa (unsweetened chocolate) powder.

Muesli Cookies

Some muesli mixes contain added milk powder so do check the label.

MAKES ABOUT 30

75 g/3 oz/⅓ cup soya spread

75 g/3 oz/⅓ cup light brown sugar

25 ml/1½ tbsp golden (light corn) syrup

5 ml/1 tsp bicarbonate of soda (baking soda)

75 g/3 oz/¾ cup plain (all-purpose) flour

150 g/5 oz/1¼ cups muesli

Oil, for greasing

1 Melt the soya spread, sugar and syrup in a saucepan.

2 Add the bicarbonate of soda – the mixture will froth. Stir in the flour and muesli.

3 Shape into walnut-sized balls and place a little apart on two greased baking (cookie) sheets.

4 Flatten slightly with a fork. Bake in a preheated oven at 190°C/375°F/gas mark 5 for about 10 minutes until golden.

5 Leave to cool for a few minutes, then transfer to a wire rack to cool completely. Store in an airtight container.

Ginger Crumblies

100 g/4 oz/½ cup soya spread

100 g/4 oz/½ cup caster (superfine) sugar

225 g/8 oz/2 cups plain (all-purpose) flour

30 ml/2 tbsp ground ginger

5 ml/1 tsp baking powder

1 small egg, beaten

Pieces of crystallised (candied) ginger, to decorate

1 Put all the ingredients in a food processor and run the machine until the mixture forms a ball.

2 Shape into a roll about 5 cm/2 in thick and wrap in greaseproof (waxed) paper. Chill in the fridge (it will keep for up to 2 weeks) before use.

3 Cut into slices about 5 mm/¼ in thick and place on greased baking (cookie) sheet. Top each with a piece of crystallised ginger. Bake in a preheated oven at 190°C/375°F/gas mark 5 for 10–12 minutes until golden.

4 Transfer to a wire rack to cool. Store in an airtight container.

SAUCES, DRESSINGS, CHEESES AND CREAMS

Many sauces and accompaniments contain dairy products, and of course cream and many cheeses are absolutely out of the question. However, there are plenty of ideas in this section that will complement your dairy-free diet perfectly. And there are a few recipes for basic sauces that no cook can do without!

Basic White Sauce

SERVES 4

45 ml/3 tbsp plain (all-purpose) flour

300 ml/½ pt/1¼ cups soya milk

A knob of soya spread

Salt and freshly ground black pepper

1 Mix the flour with a little of the milk in a saucepan. Blend in the remaining milk and add the soya spread.

2 Bring to the boil and cook for 2 minutes, stirring, until thickened and smooth. Season to taste.

Parsley Sauce

SERVES 4

1 Prepare 1 quantity of Basic White Sauce (above).

2 Stir in 45 ml/3 tbsp chopped fresh parsley.

Mushroom Sauce

SERVES 4

1 Prepare 1 quantity of Basic White Sauce (above).

2 Chop 4–6 button mushrooms and stew in 30 ml/2 tbsp water until soft and stir into the prepared sauce.

Tip: For extra flavour, make Parsley Sauce and Mushroom Sauce using Béchamel Sauce (see page 179) instead of Basic White Sauce.

Béchamel Sauce

1 slice of onion

1 bay leaf

A few black peppercorns

300 ml/½ pt/1¼ cups soya milk

45 ml/3 tbsp plain (all-purpose) flour

A knob of soya spread

A pinch of salt

1 Put the onion, bay leaf, peppercorns and soya milk in a saucepan. Bring to the boil. Remove from the heat and leave to infuse for 15 minutes. Strain the milk and discard the flavourings.

2 Mix a little of the milk with the flour in a saucepan. Blend in the remaining milk and add the soya spread.

3 Bring to the boil and cook for 2 minutes, stirring, until thickened and smooth. Season with salt and use as required.

Tomato Sauce

SERVES 4

1 onion, finely chopped

1 garlic clove, crushed

30 ml/2 tbsp olive oil

400 g/14 oz/1 large can of chopped tomatoes

15 ml/1 tbsp tomato purée (paste)

2.5 ml/½ tsp dried basil or oregano

5 ml/1 tsp caster (superfine) sugar

Salt and freshly ground black pepper

1 Fry (sauté) the onion and garlic in the oil for 2 minutes, stirring.

2 Add all the remaining ingredients, bring to the boil, reduce the heat and simmer for about 5 minutes until pulpy.

3 Taste and adjust the seasoning, if necessary. Use as required.

Provençal Sauce

SERVES 4

1 Prepare 1 quantity of Tomato Sauce (above), adding a finely chopped green (bell) pepper with the onion and garlic.

2 Stir in 50 g/2 oz sliced, stoned (pitted) black olives before serving.

Barbecue Sauce

15 ml/1 tbsp lemon juice

15 ml/1 tbsp malt vinegar

45 ml/3 tbsp tomato ketchup (catsup)

15 ml/1 tbsp Worcestershire sauce

30 ml/2 tbsp golden (light corn) syrup or clear honey

Mix all the ingredients together and use as a dipping sauce or to brush over plain meats before grilling (broiling).

Jam Sauce

60 ml/4 tbsp any flavour jam (conserve), chopped if necessary

30 ml/2 tbsp caster (superfine) sugar

*Finely grated rind and juice of ½ lemon
or 15 ml/1 tbsp lemon juice*

75 ml/5 tbsp water

1 Put all the ingredients in a saucepan.

2 Heat gently, stirring, until melted. Simmer for 3 minutes.

3 Use as required.

Sweet White Sauce

SERVES 4

300 ml/½ pt/1¼ cups soya milk

30 ml/2 tbsp cornflour (cornstarch)

30 ml/2 tbsp caster (superfine) sugar

1 Blend a little of the milk with the cornflour in a saucepan. Stir in the remaining milk and the sugar.

2 Bring to the boil and cook for 1 minute, stirring, until thickened and smooth.

Variations

CREAMY SWEET WHITE SAUCE

1 Prepare 1 quantity of Sweet White Sauce (above) but use 250 ml/8 fl oz/1 cup of soya milk.

2 When cooked, stir in 60 ml/4 tbsp Soya Dream (see page 12).

VANILLA SAUCE

1 Prepare 1 quantity of either Sweet White Sauce or Creamy Sweet White Sauce (above).

2 Stir in a few drops of vanilla essence (extract) to taste.

CUSTARD SAUCE

1 Prepare 1 quantity of Vanilla Sauce (above).

2 Whisk in an egg yolk with the sugar before cooking.

CHOCOLATE SAUCE

1 Prepare 1 quantity of Sweet White Sauce (above).

2 Substitute half the cornflour (cornstarch) with cocoa (unsweetened chocolate) powder.

Soft Soya Cheese

The cheese will keep in the fridge for up to a week.

MAKES ABOUT 225 G/8 OZ/1 CUP

500 g/1 lb 2 oz /1 tub of soya yoghurt

1 Line a sieve (strainer) with an unused disposable kitchen cloth. Place over a bowl.

2 Tip in the yoghurt and fold the edges of the cloth over so it doesn't drip down the sides.

3 Place in the fridge for several hours or overnight.

4 Spoon the soft cheese into a container with a lid and chill until ready to use. Alternatively, freeze in two separate quantities for later use.

Soya Soft Cheese with Chives

MAKES ABOUT 100 G/4 OZ/½ CUP

100 g/4 oz/½ cup Soft Soya Cheese (above)

15 ml/1 tbsp snipped fresh chives

Salt and freshly ground black pepper

1 Mix the cheese with the chives and season to taste.

2 Tip into an airtight container. Chill for at least 30 minutes to allow the flavours to develop. Use as required.

Soft Cheese with Garlic and Herbs

100 g/4 oz/½ cup Soft Soya Cheese (see page 183)

1 small garlic clove, crushed

15 ml/1 tbsp chopped fresh parsley

2.5 ml/½ tsp dried mixed herbs

Salt and freshly ground black pepper

1 Mix the cheese with the garlic and herbs and season to taste.

2 Chill for at least 30 minutes to allow the flavours to develop.

Cheesy Spread

Flavour this as you wish with chopped bacon, garlic, herbs, etc. It can be used like ordinary cheese spread and can even be melted on toast.

MAKES ABOUT 100 G/4 OZ/½ CUP

50 g/2 oz/¼ cup Soft Soya Cheese (see page 183)

50 g/2 oz/¼ cup soya spread

15 ml/1 tbsp full-fat soya flour

A good pinch of salt

A few drops of lemon juice

1 Beat together the Soft Soya Cheese and soya spread thoroughly until completely blended, then beat in the salt and soya flour. Sharpen very slightly with lemon juice, to taste.

2 Line a ramekin dish (custard cup) with kitchen paper (paper towels), then a fairly large piece of greaseproof (waxed) paper.

3 Pack the cheese spread into the pot and fold the paper over the top to cover completely. Top this with a double thickness of kitchen paper, folded to fit in the top.

4 Place a small plastic lid or a sheet of card that will just fit inside the dish on top and weight down with heavy weights. Chill for at least 24 hours, preferably 48 hours. Remove from the dish, unwrap and store in an airtight container. Use as required.

Soya 'Whipped Cream'

MAKES ABOUT 300 ML/½ PT/1¼ CUPS

5 ml/1 tsp powdered gelatine

15 ml/1 tbsp water

150 ml/¼ pt/⅔ cup Soya Dream (see page 12), chilled

A little caster (superfine) sugar (optional)

1 Put the gelatine in a small bowl and stir in the water. Stand the bowl in a pan of gently simmering water and stir until the gelatine is completely dissolved.

2 Whisk the Soya Dream in a bowl with an electric beater until thick and almost doubled in bulk. Sweeten to taste, if liked, with sugar.

3 Whisk in the gelatine, then place the mixture in the fridge for about 30 minutes to set. Use as required instead of whipped cream.

Almond Cream

Use this as a topping for desserts – it's delicious on everything from steamed sponges to fresh fruit salad. Try making it with ground hazelnuts (filberts) for a change, too.

SERVES 4

50 g/2 oz/½ cup ground almonds

60 ml/4 tbsp cold water

10 ml/2 tsp caster (superfine) sugar

Blend the nuts with the water and sugar to a soft, dropping consistency. Use as required.

INDEX

allergies 7, 10
almond cream 186
almost tiramisu 132
American pork 'n' beans 104–105
anaphylactic shock 10
anchovies
  bruschetta 52
apples
  toffee apples 153
  tofu apple and blackberry kissel 25
apricot fool 125
artichokes
  beef stroganoff with artichokes 92
asparagus
  smoked tofu with asparagus
    stir-fry 86
aubergines
  aubergine and red pepper soup
    with rouille 46–47
  aubergine dip with crudités 54
babies
  cows' milk protein allergy 10
bacon
  bacon and bean quiche 97
  green pea and bacon soup 44
  herby mushroom and egg cups
    with crunchy bacon 32–33
  potato cakes with bacon and
    eggs 31
baked beans
  bacon and bean quiche 97
baked gammon with potato cake
  102–103
bananas
  banana breakfast whip 24
  banana condé 133
  banana, strawberry and almond
    wake-up 24
  chocolate smoothie 156
  spiced banana and corn toppers 51
barbecue sauce 181
basic bread dough 158
basic white sauce 178
beans see individual types
béchamel sauce 179
beef
  beef stroganoff with artichokes 92
  very slow-cooked braised beef in
    red wine 88–89
  see also beef (minced); steak
beef (minced)
  crispy beef pancakes 139
  rich weekday mince with baby
    vegetables 91
biscuits
  chocolate digestives 151
  chocolate fork biscuits 174
  digestive biscuits 150

fork biscuits 174
ginger crumblies 176
gingerbread men 152–153
muesli cookies 175
Black Forest gâteau 166
blueberries
  fresh blueberry muffins 38
bread
  basic bread dough 158
  bread and jam pudding 122
  brioches 34–35
  crusty loaf 159
  doughnut bites 124
  garlic bread 161
  herb and sunflower seed bread 163
  milk bread 160
  quick sun-dried tomato and olive
    rolls 162
  quick walnut rolls 163
  soya breakfast rolls 37
breakfasts 23
  banana breakfast whip 24
  banana, strawberry and almond
    wake-up 24
  breakfast compôte 26
  brioches 34–35
  creamy golden trickle porridge 28
  English breakfast muffins 36–37
  French toast 35
  fresh blueberry muffins 38
  herby mushroom and egg cups
    with crunchy bacon 32–33
  honey fruit and nut crunch 27
  kipper and egg scramble 33
  potato cakes with bacon and
    eggs 31
  soya breakfast rolls 37
  summer porridge 30
  tofu apple and blackberry kissel 25
  Tropical oats 29
breastfeeding 10
brioches 34–35
bruschetta 52
bulgar wheat
  monkfish tabbouleh 62–63
butter alternatives 12
buttery crispy popcorn 155
cakes
  Black Forest gâteau 166
  chocolate cream buns 146
  cinnamon ring doughnuts 148
  dark chocolate balls 144
  everyday fruit cake 167
  jam and 'cream' sponge 165
  jam doughnuts 147
  maids of honour 171
  marshmallow dream cake 149
  see also biscuits; scones

calcium 16
carbohydrates 15
carrot and cumin soup 42
cashew nuts
  trout with cashew nuts 63
cheese 10
  alternatives to 12
  cheese and tomato pizza 138
  cheesy spread 185
  soft cheese with garlic and
    herbs 184
  soft soya cheese 183
  soya soft cheese with chives 183
cheesecakes
  lemon cheesecake 123
cheesy spread 185
cherries with kirsch zabaglione 134
chicken
  chicken and corn chowder 45
  chicken dippers 140
  chicken satay with fresh
    pineapple 110–111
  mini Kievs 141
  oven-fried chicken and potatoes
    with sour chive dip 116–117
  smoky Caesar salad 112–113
  South Pacific chicken 118
  stuffed pot roast chicken 114–115
chickpeas
  ratatouille with chickpeas and
    eggs 82–83
children
  allergies 7
children's specials
  buttery crispy popcorn 155
  cheese and tomato pizza 138
  chicken dippers 140
  chocolate cream buns 146
  chocolate digestives 151
  chocolate smoothie 156
  cinnamon ring doughnuts 148
  crispy beef pancakes 139
  dark chocolate balls 144
  digestive biscuits 150
  funky fish cakes 142–143
  gingerbread men 152–153
  jam doughnuts 147
  knickerbocker glory 145
  marshmallow dream cake 149
  mini Kievs 141
  sizzling peanut pizza 139
  teacup honey fluff nougat 154–155
  toffee apples 153
chocolate
  chocolate cream buns 146
  chocolate digestives 151
  chocolate fork biscuits 174
  chocolate ice 121
  chocolate sauce 182
  chocolate smoothie 156
  dark chocolate balls 144
  profiteroles with dark chocolate
    spread 135

choux pastry 170
chowders see soup
cinnamon ring doughnuts 148
coffee ice 121
commercial food products 12–13
confectionery
  buttery crispy popcorn 155
  dark chocolate balls 144
  teacup honey fluff nougat 154–155
  toffee apples 153
corn see sweetcorn
cows' milk
  importance in diet 11
cows' milk protein allergy 7, 10
crab and cucumber gougère 65
cream
  alternatives 12
  almond cream 186
  soya 'whipped cream' 186
creamy golden trickle porridge 28
creamy mushroom soup 40
creamy sweet white sauce 182
crème brûlée 127
crispy beef pancakes 139
crostini with olives and
  mushrooms 53
crusty loaf 159
curry turnovers 108–109
custard sauce 182
dairy products
  alternatives to 11–12, 15, 17
  importance in diet 11
dark chocolate balls 144
desserts
  almost tiramisu 132
  apricot fool 125
  banana condé 133
  Black Forest gâteau 166
  bread and jam pudding 122
  cherries with kirsch zabaglione 134
  chocolate cream buns 146
  crème brûlée 127
  dark chocolate balls 144
  doughnut bites 124
  flavoured ice creams 121
  Greek-style yoghurt with
    figs 130
  hazelnut Pavlova with
    raspberries 128
  knickerbocker glory 145
  lemon cheesecake 123
  peach filo tarts 126
  pear brûlée 131
  profiteroles with dark chocolate
    spread 135
  simple pancakes 173
  toffee orange greengage
    pudding 129
  vanilla ice 120
diet 15–16
  seven-day plan 19–21
digestive biscuits 150
  chocolate digestives 151

dips
    aubergine dip with crudités 54
    see also sauces
doughnuts
    cinnamon ring doughnuts 148
    doughnut bites 124
    jam doughnuts 147
drinks
    banana breakfast whip 24
    banana, strawberry and almond
        wake-up 24
    chocolate smoothie 156
eggs
    French toast 35
    herby mushroom and egg cups
        with crunchy bacon 32–33
    kipper and egg scramble 33
    potato cakes with bacon and
        eggs 31
    ratatouille with chickpeas and
        eggs 82–83
    savoury egg pasta 74–75
English breakfast muffins 36–37
everyday fruit cake 167
exercise 16
fajitas
    spicy prawn fajitas 70–71
fats 15–16
fibre 15
figs
    Greek-style yoghurt with figs 130
filo pastry
    peach filo tarts 126
    pork and prawn spring rolls with
        egg fried rice 106–107
    salmon in filo pastry 69
fish 61
    funky fish cakes 142–143
    tandoori fish with tomato and
        mango rice 66–67
    see also individual types
flageolet beans
    rich lamb and bean hot-pot 93
flaky pastry 169
food
    allergies 7
    commercially produced 12–14
fork biscuits 174
French toast 35
fresh blueberry muffins 38
fruit 15
    breakfast compôte 26
    fresh blueberry muffins 38
    fruit ice 121
    fruit ripple 121
    fruit scones 164
    summer porridge 30
    see also individual types
funky fish cakes 142–143
gammon
    baked gammon with potato
        cake 102–103
garlic bread 161

ginger crumblies 176
gingerbread men 152–153
goats' milk 12
gougère
    crab and cucumber gougère 65
Greek-style yoghurt with figs 130
green pea and bacon soup 44
greengages
    toffee orange greengage
        pudding 129
grilled marinated tofu on toast 55
grilled salmon with watercress
    hollandaise 68
haricot beans
    American pork 'n' beans 104–105
hazelnut Pavlova with
    raspberries 128
herb and sunflower seed bread 163
herby mushroom and egg cups with
    crunchy bacon 32–33
honey fruit and nut crunch 27
hot sweet and sour ribs 98–99
ice cream 120–121
jam and 'cream' sponge 165
jam doughnuts 147
jam sauce 181
kipper and egg scramble 33
knickerbocker glory 145
lactase 9
lactose
    hidden in commercial
        products 12–14
    intolerance 7, 9–10
lamb
    Moroccan lamb 94–95
    red lamb with rosemary 96
    rich lamb and bean hot-pot 93
leeks
    velvet leek and potato soup 49
lemon cheesecake 123
lentils
    lentil and tomato soup with
        cardamom 48
    spicy lentil and chestnut
        mushroom rissoles 76–77
lunches *see* starters and snacks
mackerel
    smoked mackerel and potato
        bowls 64
maids of honour 171
margarine alternatives 12
marshmallow dream cake 149
medicines 14
melon
    pale green dream 50
mighty minestrone 43
milk
    alternatives 11–12, 17
    hidden in commercial
        products 12–14
    milk bread 160
    see also cows' milk; soya milk
milk products 12–14

minerals 15
minestrone
  mighty minestrone 43
mini Kievs 141
monkfish tabbouleh 62–63
Moroccan lamb 94–95
muesli cookies 175
muffins
  English breakfast muffins 36–37
  fresh blueberry muffins 38
mushrooms
  creamy mushroom soup 40
  crostini with olives and
    mushrooms 53
  herby mushroom and egg cups
    with crunchy bacon 32–33
  mushroom sauce 178
  spicy lentil and chestnut
    mushroom rissoles 76–77
  tagliatelle with pesto and oyster
    mushrooms 81
noodles
  very slow-cooked braised beef in
    red wine 88–89
nougat
  teacup honey fluff nougat 154–155
oven-fried chicken and potatoes
  with sour chive dip 116–117
pale green dream 50
pancakes
  crispy beef pancakes 139
  simple pancakes 173
parsley sauce 178
pasta
  savoury egg pasta 74–75
  tagliatelle with pesto and oyster
    mushrooms 81
  very slow-cooked braised beef in
    red wine 88–89
pastry
  choux 170
  flaky 169
  shortcrust 168
pastry dishes
  bacon and bean quiche 97
  chocolate cream buns 146
  crab and cucumber gougère 65
  curry turnovers 108–109
  maids of honour 171
  peach filo tarts 126
  pissaladière 72–73
  pork and prawn spring rolls with
    egg fried rice 106–107
  profiteroles with dark chocolate
    spread 135
  salmon in filo pastry 69
pâtés
  sardine pâté crispers 56
peach filo tarts 126
peanut butter
  peanut rarebit 57
  sizzling peanut pizza 139
pear brûlée 131

peas
  green pea and bacon soup 44
peppers
  aubergine and red pepper soup
    with rouille 46–47
pilchard pots 58
pissaladière 72–73
pizzas
  cheese and tomato pizza 138
  sizzling peanut pizza 139
plain yoghurt scones 164
popcorn
  buttery crispy popcorn 155
pork
  American pork 'n' beans 104–105
  hot sweet and sour ribs 98–99
  pork and prawn spring rolls with
    egg fried rice 106–107
  see also bacon; gammon
porridge
  creamy golden trickle
    porridge 28
  summer porridge 30
potatoes
  baked gammon with potato
    cake 102–103
  potato cakes with bacon and
    eggs 31
  smoked mackerel and potato
    bowls 64
  velvet leek and potato soup 49
prawns
  pork and prawn spring rolls with
    egg fried rice 106–107
  spicy prawn fajitas 70–71
profiteroles with dark chocolate
  spread 135
proteins 15
Provençal sauce 180
quiches
  bacon and bean quiche 97
quick sun-dried tomato and olive
  rolls 162
quick walnut rolls 163
Quorn 15
raspberries
  hazelnut Pavlova with
    raspberries 128
ratatouille with chickpeas and
  eggs 82–83
red lamb with rosemary 96
ribs
  hot sweet and sour ribs 98–99
rice
  rice and vegetable stir-fry 80
  soya bean roast with curried rice
    salad 84–85
  tandoori fish with tomato and
    mango rice 66–67
rich lamb and bean hot-pot 93
rich tomato and rice soup 41
rich weekday mince with baby
  vegetables 91

rissoles
  spicy lentil and chestnut
    mushroom rissoles 76–77
rolls
  quick sun-dried tomato and olive
    rolls 162
  quick walnut rolls 163
  soya breakfast rolls 37
roulades
  spinach and sweetcorn
    roulade 78–79
sage and onion sausage toad with
  carrot gravy 100–101
salads
  smoky Caesar salad 112–113
salmon
  grilled salmon with watercress
    hollandaise 68
  salmon in filo pastry 69
sardine pâté crispers 56
satay
  chicken satay with fresh
    pineapple 110–111
sauces
  barbecue sauce 181
  basic white sauce 178
  béchamel sauce 179
  chocolate sauce 182
  creamy sweet white sauce 182
  custard sauce 182
  jam sauce 181
  mushroom sauce 178
  parsley sauce 178
  Provençal sauce 180
  sweet white sauce 182
  tomato sauce 180
  vanilla sauce 182
sausages
  sage and onion sausage toad with
    carrot gravy 100–101
savoury egg pasta 74–75
scones
  fruit scones 164
  plain yoghurt scones 164
  sweet yoghurt scones 164
sheeps' milk 12
shortcrust pastry 168
simple pancakes 173
sizzling peanut pizza 139
smoked mackerel and potato
  bowls 64
smoked tofu with asparagus
  stir-fry 86
smoky Caesar salad 112–113
snacks see starters and snacks
soft cheese with garlic and
  herbs 184
soft soya cheese 183
soup 39
  aubergine and red pepper soup
    with rouille 46–47
  carrot and cumin soup 42
  chicken and corn chowder 45

creamy mushroom soup 40
green pea and bacon soup 44
lentil and tomato soup with
  cardamom 48
mighty minestrone 43
rich tomato and rice soup 41
velvet leek and potato soup 49
South Pacific chicken 118
soya bean roast with curried rice
  salad 84–85
soya breakfast rolls 37
Soya Dream 12
soya milk 11, 17
  banana breakfast whip 24
  banana, strawberry and almond
    wake-up 24
soya soft cheese with chives 183
soya spread 12
soya 'whipped cream' 186
soya yoghurt 12
spiced banana and corn toppers 51
spicy lentil and chestnut mushroom
  rissoles 76–77
spicy prawn fajitas 70–71
spinach and sweetcorn roulade 78–79
starch 15
starters and snacks 39
  aubergine dip with crudités 54
  bruschetta 52
  crostini with olives and
    mushrooms 53
  grilled marinated tofu on toast 55
  pale green dream 50
  peanut rarebit 57
  pilchard pots 58
  sardine pâté crispers 56
  spiced banana and corn toppers 51
  tofu cakes 59
steak
  steak strips sizzle with crunchy
    noodles 90
stir-fries
  rice and vegetable stir-fry 80
  smoked tofu with asparagus
    stir-fry 86
stuffed pot roast chicken 114–115
sugars 15
summer porridge 30
suppers see starters
Swedish oat drink 11
sweet white sauce 182
sweet yoghurt scones 164
sweetcorn
  chicken and corn chowder 45
  spiced banana and corn
    toppers 51
  spinach and sweetcorn
    roulade 78–79
sweets see confectionery
tabbouleh
  monkfish tabbouleh 62–63
tagliatelle with pesto and oyster
  mushrooms 81

tandoori fish with tomato and
    mango rice 66–67
teacup honey fluff nougat 154–155
tiramisu
    almost tiramisu 132
toffee apples 153
toffee orange greengage pudding 129
tofu 12, 15
    grilled marinated tofu on toast 55
    smoked tofu with asparagus
        stir-fry 86
    tofu apple and blackberry kissel 25
    tofu cakes 59
tomatoes
    rich tomato and rice soup 41
    tomato sauce 180
Tropical oats 29
trout with cashew nuts 63
vanilla ice 120
vanilla sauce 182

vegetables 15, 61
    ratatouille with chickpeas and
        eggs 82–83
    rice and vegetable stir-fry 80
    rich weekday mince with baby
        vegetables 91
    see also individual types
velvet leek and potato soup 49
very slow-cooked braised beef in red
    wine 88–89
vitamins 15
watercress
    grilled salmon with watercress
        hollandaise 68
yoghurt (soya) 12
    Greek-style yoghurt with figs 130
    sweet yoghurt scones 164
Yorkshire pudding 172
zabaglione
    cherries with kirsch zabaglione 134